Diverticulitis Cookbook For Beginners

From Pain to Comfort with 2000+ Recipes, a 3-Phase Diet Guide, Essential Flare-Up Management Strategies, and an Exclusive Life-Saving Emergency Plan

Dr. Madison Wells

Table Of Content

Table Of Content	2
Introduction	8
Chapter 1: Understanding Diverticulitis	10
1.1 The Basics of Diverticulitis: What You Need to Know	10
1.2 The Role of Diet in Managing Diverticulitis	11
Foods to Include	11
Foods to Avoid	12
Tips	12
Takeaway	12
1.3 Recognizing Symptoms and Identifying Flare-Ups	13
Symptom Recognition:	13
Identifying Flare-Ups:	13
Your Healing Journey:	13
1.4 The Importance of a Balanced Gut: Insights into Fiber, Flora, and Your Health	14
The Role of Fiber in Bowel Regularity and Diverticulitis Management	14
Insights into the Dynamic Influence of Gut Flora on Your Health	14
Unveiling the Symbiotic Relationship between Fiber and Gut Flora	15
Chapter 2: The Diverticulitis Healing Journey	16
2.1 Phases of Diverticulitis: An Overview	16
Stage 1: Diverticulosis - Silent Presence of Pouches	16
Stage 2: Diverticulitis Flare-ups - Acute Inflammation and Symptoms	16
Stage 3: Complicated Diverticulitis - Severe Infection and Complications	16
Dietary Strategies Across Diverticulitis Phases - Nurturing Your Gut Health	17
Empower Your Healing Journey Through Nutrition	17
2.2 Personalizing Your Diet: How to Tailor Your Food Choices to Your Needs	17
Embracing Personalization: Your Unique Dietary Pathway	17
Phase-Specific Dietary Guidance: Navigating Diverticulosis, Flare-Ups, and Complications	18
In Diverticulosis: Nurturing Your Gut Health	18
During Flare-Ups: Easing Discomfort and Reducing Irritation	18
In Complicated Diverticulitis: Prioritizing Healing and Well-Being	18
Tailoring Your Diet: Practical Tips and Recipe Guidance	19
Ingredient Selection: Prioritizing Nourishment and Digestive Comfort	19
Meal Planning: Creating Balanced and Flavorful Meals	19
Exploring Easy-to-Follow Recipes: Accessible, Nutrient-Dense Delights	19
Empowerment Through Personalized Nutrition	19
2.3 Monitoring Symptoms and Dietary Reactions	20
Tuning In: Listening to Your Body	20
Identifying Trigger Foods and Lifestyle Factors	20

Working with Healthcare Professionals	21
Adjusting Your Diet Based on Observations	21
The Power of Data: Tracking Your Progress	22
Staying Empowered and Informed	22
2.4 Stress and Its Impact on Diverticulitis: Managing More Than Just Your Diet	22
The Stress-Diverticulitis Connection	22
Coping with Stress: Strategies for Diverticulitis Management	23
The Importance of a Holistic Approach	24
Next Steps: Moving Forward with Confidence	24
Chapter 3: Dietary Foundations for Diverticulitis	**25**
3.1 Safe Foods: Building Your Diverticulitis-Friendly Pantry	25
Diverticulitis and Safe Foods	25
Creating Diverticulitis-Friendly Meals	26
3.2 Foods to Avoid: Understanding Potential Triggers	27
The Problematic Culprits: Foods to Stay Away From	27
1. High-Fiber Foods	27
2. Nuts and Seeds	27
3. Spicy Foods	28
4. Caffeine and Alcohol	28
Navigating the Elimination Process: A Step-by-Step Approach	28
3.3 The Importance of Hydration: Best Practices for Fluid Intake	29
The Role of Hydration in Digestive Health	30
Empowering Your Hydration Journey	31
3.4 Balancing Nutrients: Proteins, Fats, and Carbohydrates	32
Proteins: Building Blocks for Health	32
Fats: The Right Choices for Optimal Health	32
Carbohydrates: Fuel for Energy	33
Striking the Balance: Practical Tips	33
Practical Examples	34
Chapter 4: Recipes for Relief and Recovery	**35**
4.1 Breakfast Recipes: A Gentle Start to Your Day	35
Nourishing Morning Meals	35
Guidelines for Digestive-Friendly Breakfasts	35
4.1.1 Smoothies and Juices: Nutrient-Dense Morning Boosters	36
4.1.2 Porridge and Warm Cereals: Soothing Whole Grain Options	37
4.1.3 Egg Dishes: Protein-Rich Breakfasts with a Gentle Touch	40
4.1.4 Breakfast Breads and Pastries: Fiber-Enriched Bites for the Morning	42
4.2 Nourishing Lunches: Meals That Fuel and Heal	44
Understanding the Importance of Nourishment	45
Guidelines for Nourishing Lunches	45
Nourishing Lunch Ideas	46

    4.2.1 Salads: Colorful, Fiber-Filled Combinations ... 47
    4.2.2 Light Soups: Comforting Broths and Pureed Varieties ... 49
    4.2.3 Sandwiches and Wraps: Balanced, Digestion-Friendly Lunches ... 52
    4.2.4 Bowls: Wholesome Lunch Bowls with Digestion-Supporting Ingredients ... 54
4.3 Dinners for Optimal Gut Health ... 56
    4.3.1 Grilled and Baked Proteins: Gentle and Satisfying Main Courses ... 57
    4.3.2 Vegetable Sides: Steamed and Roasted Options for Gut Health ... 59
    4.3.3 Casseroles: One-Dish Meals Made with Ease ... 61
    4.3.4 Stir-Fries: Quick and Customizable for a Gentle Evening Meal ... 63
4.4 Snacks and Mini-Meals: Eating Well Between Meals ... 65
    The Essential Role of Snacks and Mini-Meals ... 65
    Hummus – the Wholesome Dip ... 65
    Invincible Smoothies: Tailor-made Nutrition in a Glass ... 65
    Broths to Boost Wellness ... 66
    Optimizing Popcorn for Diverticulitis ... 66
    4.4.1 Healthy Fats and Nuts: Small Portions for Sustained Energy ... 66
    4.4.2 Fruit-Based Snacks: Gentle on the Digestive System ... 68
    4.4.3 Homemade Bars and Energy Balls: Nutrient-Packed Bites ... 71
    4.4.4 Yogurts and Probiotic-Rich Foods: Supporting Gut Flora ... 73
4.5 Special Section: International Cuisine Diverticulitis-Friendly Dishes ... 75
    4.5.1 Asian-Inspired Recipes: Flavorful Dishes with a Digestive Twist ... 77
    4.5.2 Mediterranean Delights: Heart-Healthy Fats and Grains ... 79
    4.5.3 Latin American Fare: Mild Yet Robust Flavor Profiles ... 81
    4.5.4 European Classics: Comforting Meals Reimagined for Gut Health ... 83

Chapter 5: Meal Planning and Preparation ... **88**
5.1 Creating a Diverticulitis Meal Plan: A Week's Worth of Ideas ... 88
    Understanding Your Dietary Needs ... 88
    Day 1: Kick-Start Your Week ... 88
    Day 2: Midweek Boost ... 88
    Day 3: Variety Is Key ... 88
    Day 4: Savory Delights ... 89
    Day 5: Fresh and Flavorful ... 89
    Day 6: Simple Pleasures ... 89
    Day 7: Satisfying End to the Week ... 89
5.2 Meal Prep Strategies for Busy Lifestyles ... 89
    Simplify Your Ingredients ... 89
    Batch Cooking for Efficiency ... 90
    Strategic Snack Planning ... 90
    Embrace Make-Ahead Meals ... 90
    Utilize Time-Saving Kitchen Tools ... 90
    Customize Your Meal Prep Routine ... 90

5.3 Shopping and Ingredient Swaps: Navigating the Grocery Store — 91
- Understanding Your Grocery Store Environment — 91
- Embracing Fresh, Wholesome Ingredients — 91
- Making Smart Ingredient Swaps — 91
- Reading Labels and Making Informed Choices — 92
- Building a Diverse and Balanced Pantry — 92
- Seeking Guidance from Health Professionals — 92

Chapter 6: Lifestyle Modification and Additional Tips — 93

6.1 Exercise and Diverticulitis: What You Need to Know — 93
- The Benefits of Exercise for Diverticulitis Management — 93
- Choosing the Right Exercise for Diverticulitis — 93
- Tips for Incorporating Exercise into your Routine — 94

6.2 The Mind-Gut Connection: Understanding How Stress Affects Symptoms — 95
- The Mind-Gut Connection: Explained — 95
- How Stress Affects Diverticulitis Symptoms — 95
- Stress Management Techniques for Diverticulitis — 96

6.3 Building Your Support System: Family, Friends, and Online Communities — 97
- The Power of Familial Support — 97
- Embracing Supportive friendships — 97
- The Benefits of Online Communities — 97
- Nurturing Your Support Network — 98
- Empowerment through Collective Strength — 98

Conclusion — 99
- The Power of Knowledge and Confidence — 99
- Navigating Dietary Choices with Precision — 99
- Harmonizing Flavors and Textures — 99
- Embracing Culinary Creativity — 99
- Savoring the Journey Ahead — 100
- Empowerment Through Culinary Mastery — 100
- Empowering Your Culinary Legacy — 100

© Copyright 2024 by Dr. Madison Wells - All rights reserved.

The following Book is reproduced below with the goal of providing information that is as accurate and reliable as possible. Regardless, purchasing this Book can be seen as consent to the fact that both the publisher and the author of this book are in no way experts on the topics discussed within and that any recommendations or suggestions that are made herein are for entertainment purposes only. Professionals should be consulted as needed prior to undertaking any of the action endorsed herein.

This declaration is deemed fair and valid by both the American Bar Association and the Committee of Publishers Association and is legally binding throughout the United States.

Furthermore, the transmission, duplication, or reproduction of any of the following work including specific information will be considered an illegal act irrespective of if it is done electronically or in print. This extends to creating a secondary or tertiary copy of the work or a recorded copy and is only allowed with the express written consent from the Publisher. All additional rights reserved.

The information in the following pages is broadly considered a truthful and accurate account of facts and as such, any inattention, use, or misuse of the information in question by the reader will render any resulting actions solely under their purview. There are no scenarios in which the publisher or the original author of this work can be in any fashion deemed liable for any hardship or damages that may befall them after undertaking information described herein.

Additionally, the information in the following pages is intended only for informational purposes and should thus be thought of as universal. As befitting its nature, it is presented without assurance regarding its prolonged validity or interim quality. Trademarks that are mentioned are done without written consent and can in no way be considered an endorsement from the trademark holder.

Introduction

Welcome to "Diverticulitis Cookbook for Beginners". If you've recently been diagnosed with diverticulitis or have been battling the condition for some time, you're likely seeking reassurance, clear guidance, and practical solutions to help manage your symptoms and maintain a balanced, enjoyable diet. Through this comprehensive guide, I aim to equip you with not only reliable information about diverticulitis management but also an array of flavorful, easy-to-prepare recipes to help you feel in control of your health while enjoying delicious, gut-friendly meals.

In this book, you'll find concrete information about understanding diverticulitis, managing symptoms through diet, and the crucial role of a balanced gut in your overall health. Together, we'll explore how to personalize your dietary choices, effectively plan and prepare meals, while also addressing the impact of stress and lifestyle modifications on your condition.

As someone who values clear explanations and trustworthy information, you'll appreciate the detailed dietary foundations that are aimed at helping you make informed choices. This book offers practical insight into safe foods to stock in your pantry, foods to avoid, and the significance of hydration and nutrient balance. Specifically, the recipes included cater to realistic portion sizes, leverage easily accessible ingredients, and are accompanied by appetizing photos to inspire and guide you through your culinary journey.

With an overarching focus on empowering you to take charge of your diverticulitis management and reduce any anxiety surrounding food choices, this cookbook also addresses the need for convenient measurements in American and metric units. Ultimately, my goal is to ensure that you have the tools and knowledge to maintain a balanced, enjoyable diet without sacrificing flavor or exacerbating uncomfortable symptoms. Let's embark on this journey together, where you'll find not just a cookbook, but a reliable and supportive resource for enhancing your overall well-being.

Special Bonus

At the dawn of your diverticulitis management journey, I am delighted to introduce an indispensable bonus that not only enriches the content of this book but also serves as a vital companion in your quest for digestive wellness. The "Diverticulitis Flare-Up Emergency Kit" is a treasure trove of essential resources and expert guidance tailored to help you navigate the challenges of flare-ups with resilience and confidence. This bonus material, carefully curated to complement the core teachings of this book, offers a comprehensive toolkit to empower you in times of uncertainty and discomfort. By scanning the QR code provided, you can unlock a wealth of invaluable information, practical tips, and strategies designed to support you through the intricacies of diverticulitis flare-ups. Embrace this bonus resource as a beacon of knowledge and assurance, enhancing your ability to face the unpredictable nature of diverticulitis with grace and proficiency. As you delve into the depths of this supplementary material, may you find solace in knowing that you are well-equipped to address any flare-up that comes your way, bolstered by the wisdom and practical tools encapsulated in the "Diverticulitis Flare-Up Emergency kit

Chapter 1: Understanding Diverticulitis

1.1 The Basics of Diverticulitis: What You Need to Know

If you or someone you know has been recently diagnosed with diverticulitis, or has been managing the condition for some time, it's essential to gain a clear understanding of the condition. Diverticulitis refers to the inflammation or infection of small pouches, called diverticula, that can develop along the walls of the digestive tract, particularly in the colon. These pouches can become inflamed or infected due to various factors, leading to a range of uncomfortable symptoms such as abdominal pain, bloating, and changes in bowel habits, including constipation or diarrhea. Through reliable information and practical guidance, this chapter aims to provide you with clear insights into understanding diverticulitis and how to manage it effectively through diet and lifestyle modifications.

Understanding the Condition

Let's begin by understanding the basics of diverticulitis. These small pouches, known as diverticula, are usually formed due to weak areas in the colon wall, often due to increased pressure from straining during bowel movements. They can occur anywhere in the digestive tract, but they are most commonly found in the colon. When these pouches become inflamed or infected, the condition known as diverticulitis arises. There are various factors that can contribute to the development of diverticulitis, such as a low-fiber diet, sedentary lifestyle, obesity, and aging.

Addressing the Need for Dietary Management

For individuals dealing with diverticulitis, adopting appropriate dietary modifications plays a crucial role in managing the condition and preventing flare-ups. While there is a wealth of information available online, it is essential to seek reliable and accurate guidance. This chapter aims to debunk myths and clarify uncertainties surrounding the diet for diverticulitis, providing you with trustworthy advice to help you make informed food choices. By the end of this section, you will have a comprehensive understanding of the condition, its triggers, and the role of diet in managing diverticulitis, empowering you to take control of your health and well-being.

Through this chapter, we seek to provide a thorough understanding of diverticulitis, clarifying misconceptions and offering clear guidance on dietary modifications. It aims to equip you with the knowledge and confidence needed to navigate your diverticulitis management effectively.

1.2 The Role of Diet in Managing Diverticulitis

Managing diverticulitis requires a comprehensive approach that encompasses many facets of your life, including your diet. Since a primary cause of diverticulitis is the formation of small pouches called diverticula in the lining of your colon, dietary changes can reduce inflammation and prevent infection. Focusing on a healthy diet can also help you avoid triggering painful flare-ups and increase your overall quality of life.

Here, we will discuss what foods to eat and what foods to avoid and give you practical tips to tailor your eating habits to your needs.

Foods to Include

Eating a diet that is rich in fiber is essential for a healthy digestive system. Fiber, a non-digestible part of plant-based foods, provides bulk to your stool, helping it move quickly and efficiently through your intestines. This helps prevent constipation, which can cause inflammation and put strain on your diverticula. Aim for at least 25 to 35 grams of fiber each day.

Some good sources of fiber include fruits such as apples, berries, and pears, as well as vegetables such as broccoli, carrots, and spinach. Whole grains, such as brown rice, oats, and quinoa, are also fiber-rich. Legumes like lentils, black beans, and chickpeas are another excellent source of fiber. However, it is essential to note that you should start including fiber-rich foods gradually. A sudden increase in fiber intake can cause bloating and gas, which can lead to discomfort.

In addition to adding fiber, probiotics can also help manage diverticulitis symptoms. Probiotics are live bacteria found in fermented foods and supplements that can help maintain a balanced gut flora. These "good" bacteria are known for their anti-inflammatory properties, reducing the risk of infection and inflammation of your diverticula.

Foods to Avoid

Certain foods can trigger painful flare-ups of diverticulitis. It's crucial to avoid them or eat them in moderation.

Some of the most common foods to avoid include nuts and seeds, which are difficult to digest and can get stuck in your diverticula, triggering inflammation. For a long time, it was common for physicians to recommend the restriction of nuts and seeds in patients with diverticulitis. Still, current studies suggest that people with uncomplicated diverticulitis don't have to avoid nuts and seeds altogether. However, it is best to discuss your condition with your healthcare provider and a registered dietitian before adding nuts and seeds to your diet.

Processed foods and red meat also tend to trigger diverticulitis symptoms. Red meat is rich in saturated fat, which can cause inflammation throughout your body. Processed foods such as hot dogs, fast food, and potato chips, are often low in fiber and high in fat, sugar, and calories, which can worsen your diverticulitis symptoms.

Other foods to avoid in managing diverticulitis include spicy foods, alcohol, and caffeinated and carbonated drinks. Taken in large amounts, these types of foods can irritate your digestive system, leading to inflammation and infection of your diverticula.

Tips

Ease your way into a high-fiber diet. Gradually introduce more fiber-rich foods into your diet, and aim for small, frequent meals throughout the day to combat bloating and gas.

Stay hydrated. Avoiding dehydration is crucial in managing diverticulitis. Drinking enough water and other fluids helps regulate bowel movements and keep your stool soft. Aim for eight to ten cups of water a day.

Keep a food diary. Recording your meals and any food-related symptoms in a journal can help you identify specific trigger foods and evaluate the effectiveness of your diet plan.

Talk to your healthcare provider. A healthcare provider or a registered dietitian can design an individualized dietary plan specific to your needs, ensuring that you get enough fiber and nutrients from a balanced diet without triggering flare-ups.

Takeaway

Managing diverticulitis through diet is a long-term commitment that requires patience and persistence. Focusing on fiber-rich foods, probiotics, and moderate intake of trigger foods while recording your food intake and staying hydrated can help alleviate symptoms and improve your overall health. Working with healthcare providers and registered dietitians to create an individualized plan can help you gain control of your diet and minimize your risk of painful flare-ups.

1.3 Recognizing Symptoms and Identifying Flare-Ups

Upon being diagnosed with diverticulitis, it's crucial to be able to recognize the symptoms and identify potential flare-ups. Understanding your body's signals and knowing how to respond to them can greatly assist in managing the condition.

Symptom Recognition:

Symptoms of diverticulitis can vary from person to person. Common signs include abdominal pain, particularly in the lower left side, along with changes in bowel habits such as diarrhea or constipation. Some individuals may experience bloating, cramping, nausea, or fever. It's important to be attentive to these symptoms and to communicate any changes to your healthcare provider promptly.

Identifying Flare-Ups:

Recognizing flare-ups of diverticulitis is essential for those managing the condition. Flare-ups can be triggered by various factors, such as diet, stress, or other lifestyle factors. Maintaining a food diary and noting any symptoms after consuming certain foods can help identify potential triggers. Additionally, paying attention to stress levels and incorporating stress management techniques can aid in the prevention of flare-ups.

Your Healing Journey:

Throughout your journey with diverticulitis, it's important to be gentle and patient with yourself. Embracing a proactive approach to symptom recognition and flare-up management will empower you to take control of your health. By acknowledging the significance of listening to your body and understanding the impact of different factors on your symptoms, you are on the path to establishing a harmonious relationship with your condition.

In the subsequent chapters, we will delve into personalized dietary approaches, lifestyle modifications, and practical meal plans to support you on this journey toward alleviating symptoms and embracing a balanced, enjoyable diet that nurtures your overall well-being.

1.4 The Importance of a Balanced Gut: Insights into Fiber, Flora, and Your Health

Dear reader, as you embark on this insightful journey toward understanding and managing diverticulitis through dietary considerations, it is crucial to recognize the pivotal role that a balanced gut plays in promoting your overall well-being. In this section, we will delve into the significance of achieving this balance by exploring the profound impact of fiber and gut flora on your health, offering you clear, reliable insights that will empower you to make informed dietary choices and effectively manage diverticulitis.

The Role of Fiber in Bowel Regularity and Diverticulitis Management

Let's begin with an exploration of the indispensable role that fiber plays in ensuring bowel regularity, a critical factor in managing diverticulitis and minimizing the risk of painful flare-ups. Fiber, derived from various plant-based sources, serves as a foundational component in supporting healthy digestive processes. Its bulking properties aid in preventing constipation, softening stools, and promoting smoother bowel movements, all of which are essential for diverticulitis management.

Understanding the distinction between soluble and insoluble fiber enables you to make informed dietary choices that can positively impact your health. Soluble fiber, found in foods such as oats, legumes, and certain fruits, possesses the remarkable ability to dissolve in water, forming a gel-like substance in the digestive tract. This process facilitates gradual nutrient release and contributes to a sense of fullness, promoting digestive health. Conversely, insoluble fiber, prevalent in wheat bran, nuts, and many vegetables, adds bulk to the stool and facilitates its efficient passage through the digestive system.

Insights into the Dynamic Influence of Gut Flora on Your Health

Your gut microbiome, comprising a diverse community of microorganisms, plays a fundamental role in influencing various aspects of your health, making it a key player in diverticulitis management. This complex ecosystem of microorganisms impacts digestion, immune function, and overall well-being. Nurturing a healthy gut flora is essential for optimal digestive processes and bolstering your body's resilience, both of which are vital elements in managing diverticulitis.

Beneficial gut bacteria, known as probiotics, present within your gut microbiome, play a pivotal role in facilitating nutrient absorption and combating inflammation, thereby fostering a balanced internal environment. By incorporating probiotic-rich foods, such as yogurt, kefir, kimchi, and sauerkraut, into your diet, you can actively contribute to nurturing a flourishing gut microbiome and enhancing your body's resilience against diverticulitis complications.

Unveiling the Symbiotic Relationship between Fiber and Gut Flora

The interconnectedness of fiber and gut flora reveals a symbiotic relationship that holds profound implications for diverticulitis management. Fiber, acting as a prebiotic, essentially serves as nourishment for the probiotics in your gut, promoting their growth and harmonizing the various microorganisms within your digestive system. This synergy not only enhances the process of digestion but also fortifies your body's defense mechanisms, thereby fostering overall intestinal health and resilience against diverticulitis complications.

In practical terms, this understanding underscores the significance of prioritizing fiber-rich foods in your diet, such as whole grains, fruits, vegetables, and legumes. These dietary choices not only fuel the proliferation of beneficial gut bacteria but also contribute to improved digestive health and immune resilience, both of which are crucial for effectively managing diverticulitis.

Chapter 2: The Diverticulitis Healing Journey

2.1 Phases of Diverticulitis: An Overview

Dear Reader, understanding the phases of diverticulitis is essential in navigating your healing journey effectively. This condition progresses through distinct stages, each requiring specific attention and care to manage symptoms, prevent complications, and promote recovery. By familiarizing yourself with these phases, you empower yourself to make informed decisions about your diet and treatment plan, ultimately taking control of your health journey.

Stage 1: Diverticulosis - Silent Presence of Pouches

The journey begins with diverticulosis, often a silent presence in the colon characterized by the formation of small pouches (diverticula). While individuals with diverticulosis may not experience any noticeable symptoms, the presence of these pouches creates vulnerability to inflammation and infection, marking the initial phase of diverticulitis. Maintaining gut health through a fiber-rich diet is crucial during this stage, as fiber aids in preventing constipation, reducing pressure on the colon, and supporting overall digestive function, thereby minimizing the risk of diverticulitis progression.

Stage 2: Diverticulitis Flare-ups - Acute Inflammation and Symptoms

As diverticulosis progresses, some individuals may experience diverticulitis flare-ups, characterized by acute inflammation in the diverticula. Symptoms such as abdominal pain, bloating, changes in bowel movements, fever, and nausea may arise during these episodes, signaling the need for immediate attention and dietary modifications. During flare-ups, a low-fiber diet is often recommended to reduce irritation and strain on the inflamed areas, allowing the colon to heal. Incorporating easily digestible foods, such as cooked vegetables, lean proteins, and smoothies, can provide comfort and relief during this phase.

Stage 3: Complicated Diverticulitis - Severe Infection and Complications

In cases where diverticulitis is left unmanaged or becomes recurrent, complications such as abscesses, perforations, or fistulas may develop, leading to complicated diverticulitis. This stage requires prompt medical intervention, including antibiotics, possible hospitalization, and sometimes surgical procedures to address severe infection and repair damaged tissues. While medical treatment is paramount in complicated diverticulitis, maintaining a nutrient-rich diet that supports recovery and strengthens the immune system is vital. Foods high in antioxidants, vitamins, and minerals can aid in the healing process and reduce inflammation, promoting tissue repair and overall well-being.

Dietary Strategies Across Diverticulitis Phases - Nurturing Your Gut Health

Throughout the phases of diverticulitis, adopting dietary strategies tailored to each stage is key to managing symptoms, promoting healing, and preventing complications. In diverticulosis, focusing on a high-fiber diet with plenty of fruits, vegetables, whole grains, and legumes helps maintain regular bowel movements and supports digestive health. During diverticulitis flare-ups, transitioning to a low-fiber diet temporarily can ease discomfort and reduce inflammation, while including probiotic-rich foods such as yogurt and kefir can support gut health. In complicated diverticulitis, emphasizing nutrient-dense foods that aid in tissue repair and immune function is essential for recovery and long-term well-being.

Empower Your Healing Journey Through Nutrition

By understanding the distinct phases of diverticulitis and how dietary choices can influence each stage, you gain the knowledge and tools needed to empower your healing journey. Through a mindful approach to nutrition, tailored to your current phase of diverticulitis, you can take control of your health, reduce anxiety around food choices, and navigate your condition with confidence. Remember, each stage of diverticulitis presents unique challenges and opportunities for healing, and by prioritizing your well-being through nourishing, balanced meals, you set the foundation for a healthier, more vibrant tomorrow.

2.2 Personalizing Your Diet: How to Tailor Your Food Choices to Your Needs

Understanding how to personalize your diet to align with the specific needs of your diverticulitis condition is pivotal in managing symptoms, mitigating flare-ups, and regaining a sense of control over your health. This tailored approach empowers you to make informed dietary choices, reduce uncertainty about food selections, and create a well-rounded eating plan that promotes your well-being throughout different phases of diverticulitis.

Embracing Personalization: Your Unique Dietary Pathway

As someone navigating the complexities of diverticulitis, recognizing that your dietary needs are unique and evolve across the stages of the condition is crucial. Personalization begins by acknowledging that what works for one individual may not necessarily be the best approach for another. This understanding allows you to embrace your unique dietary pathway, appreciating that your food choices will be influenced by your specific symptoms, tolerance to certain foods, and the phase of diverticulitis you are currently experiencing.

Phase-Specific Dietary Guidance: Navigating Diverticulosis, Flare-Ups, and Complications

Personalizing your diet entails tailoring your food choices to the distinct phases of diverticulitis, aligning your nutrition with the specific needs of each stage.

In Diverticulosis: Nurturing Your Gut Health

During the diverticulosis phase, your focus is on nurturing your gut health and minimizing the risk of inflammation and infection in the diverticula. A high-fiber diet becomes a cornerstone of your approach, as it supports healthy bowel movements and promotes digestive wellness. Embracing an array of fruits, vegetables, whole grains, legumes, and seeds can supply the fiber needed to maintain regularity and reduce pressure on the colon, thereby supporting the prevention of diverticulitis progression.

During Flare-Ups: Easing Discomfort and Reducing Irritation

When experiencing diverticulitis flare-ups, the emphasis shifts to easing discomfort and reducing irritation in the inflamed areas of your colon. At this stage, a low-fiber diet may be recommended to alleviate strain on the digestive system and provide relief. Incorporating easily digestible foods such as cooked vegetables, ripe fruits without skin or seeds, lean proteins, and well-cooked grains can help in managing symptoms while allowing the colon to heal. Additionally, hydration becomes essential, aiding in the softening of stool and easing bowel movements.

In Complicated Diverticulitis: Prioritizing Healing and Well-Being

For those facing complicated diverticulitis, where severe infection and potential complications arise, prioritizing healing and overall well-being through nutrition becomes paramount. While medical intervention is crucial during this phase, focusing on a nutrient-dense diet rich in antioxidants, vitamins, and minerals can aid in tissue repair, strengthen the immune system, and support recovery. Incorporating foods such as colorful fruits and vegetables, lean proteins, healthy fats, and probiotic-rich sources can contribute to your healing journey, promoting overall well-being.

Tailoring Your Diet: Practical Tips and Recipe Guidance

Practical tips and recipe guidance can serve as invaluable resources in personalizing your diet for diverticulitis management. Consider the following actionable strategies to tailor your food choices:

Ingredient Selection: Prioritizing Nourishment and Digestive Comfort

Always prioritize nourishing, easily digestible ingredients, especially during flare-ups, selecting well-cooked vegetables, soft fruits, and lean proteins. Additionally, cultivating an understanding of your individual tolerance to certain foods allows you to curate a personalized list of ingredients that align with your digestive comfort and well-being.

Meal Planning: Creating Balanced and Flavorful Meals

Engaging in meal planning and preparation empowers you to integrate a variety of foods that support your diverticulitis journey. By conscientiously crafting balanced and flavorful meals that align with your dietary requirements, you can ensure that your nutritional needs are met while enjoying a diverse range of flavors and textures.

Exploring Easy-to-Follow Recipes: Accessible, Nutrient-Dense Delights

Exploring a collection of easy-to-follow recipes specifically tailored to diverticulitis management equips you with accessible, nutrient-dense delights that nourish your body and delight your palate. From comforting soups and stews to innovative grain and protein bowls, these recipes seamlessly integrate phase-specific dietary considerations while prioritizing taste and satisfaction.

Empowerment Through Personalized Nutrition

By embracing the art of personalizing your diet to meet the distinctive needs of diverticulitis, you take a vital step towards reclaiming your agency in managing your health. Tailoring your food choices to the phases of diverticulitis provides you with a sense of control, reduces anxiety around meal decisions, and fosters a balanced, enjoyable diet that supports your well-being without compromising on flavor or variety. In the journey towards empowering your diverticulitis management, personalized nutrition becomes a cornerstone, shaping your dietary pathway with practicality, wisdom, and the assurance of optimum wellness.

2.3 Monitoring Symptoms and Dietary Reactions

As you embark on your diverticulitis healing journey, it is essential to monitor your symptoms and dietary reactions closely. This vigilance will allow you to gain a deeper understanding of how different foods and lifestyle factors impact your condition, empowering you to make informed choices and effectively manage your diverticulitis.

Tuning In: Listening to Your Body

Listening to your body is a key aspect of monitoring your diverticulitis symptoms and dietary reactions. Your body communicates with you, providing valuable insights into how it responds to various foods and lifestyle factors. By paying attention to these signals, you can develop a clearer understanding of what works well for you individually.

When it comes to monitoring symptoms, be attentive to any changes or flare-ups in diverticulitis-related symptoms such as abdominal pain, bloating, changes in bowel movements, and general discomfort. Keep a journal or use a tracking app to record any patterns or triggers you notice, including specific foods that may worsen your symptoms.

Identifying Trigger Foods and Lifestyle Factors

One of the primary goals of monitoring symptoms and dietary reactions is to identify trigger foods and lifestyle factors that may exacerbate your diverticulitis symptoms. While triggers can vary from person to person, some common culprits may include:

High-Fiber Foods: While a high-fiber diet is generally encouraged for diverticulosis, some individuals may find that certain high-fiber foods can trigger symptoms during flare-ups. Pay attention to how your body responds to different types of fiber-rich foods and adjust your intake accordingly. It's important to note that this does not apply to everyone, so be mindful of your own unique reactions.

Spicy Foods: Spices, such as chili peppers and hot sauces, can be irritating to the digestive system and may worsen symptoms for some individuals. Take note of how your body reacts to spicy foods and consider reducing or eliminating them from your diet if they trigger discomfort.

Seeds and Nuts: While there is no conclusive evidence that seeds and nuts directly cause diverticulitis or complications, some individuals find that these foods can contribute to increased discomfort during flare-ups. Again, listen to your body and determine if seeds and nuts worsen your symptoms.

Alcohol and Caffeine: Alcohol and caffeine have the potential to irritate the digestive system and may lead to increased inflammation. Monitor your body's reaction to these substances and consider reducing or eliminating them from your diet if you notice a correlation between their consumption and flare-ups.

Stress and Lifestyle Factors: Stress and certain lifestyle factors, such as lack of sleep or inadequate physical activity, can impact your overall well-being, including your digestive health. It is important to recognize the influence of these factors on your diverticulitis symptoms and take steps to manage stress and prioritize a healthy lifestyle.

By diligently tracking your symptoms and identifying trigger foods and lifestyle factors, you will gain valuable insights that can guide your dietary choices and help you proactively manage your diverticulitis.

Working with Healthcare Professionals

While self-monitoring is essential, it is equally important to work collaboratively with your healthcare professionals. They possess the expertise and knowledge to provide guidance tailored to your specific condition and can help you navigate the complexities of diverticulitis.

Consult with your healthcare professional to discuss your symptoms, dietary reactions, and any concerns or questions you may have. They may recommend additional tests or examinations to gain further insights into your condition. This partnership with your healthcare team ensures that you receive comprehensive care and support on your diverticulitis healing journey.

Adjusting Your Diet Based on Observations

As you monitor your symptoms and dietary reactions, you will likely start to identify patterns and gain a deeper understanding of how specific foods affect your condition. Armed with this knowledge, you can make informed decisions about adjusting your diet to better manage your diverticulitis.

For example, if you notice that certain high-fiber foods cause discomfort during flare-ups, you might choose to temporarily reduce your fiber intake until symptoms subside. This could involve switching to cooked vegetables and well-cooked grains instead of raw or high-fiber varieties. Similarly, if you find that spicy foods worsen your symptoms, you can opt for milder flavors or alternatives that are easier on your digestive system.

Remember that the goal is not to completely eliminate entire food groups unless specifically advised by your healthcare professional, but rather to identify and avoid individual trigger foods that worsen your symptoms. This personalized approach allows you to create a well-balanced diet that supports your diverticulitis management while still enjoying a wide range of delicious and nutritious foods.

The Power of Data: Tracking Your Progress

As you continue monitoring your symptoms and dietary reactions, documenting your progress becomes an invaluable tool. Regularly reviewing your journal or tracking app entries gives you a detailed overview of how changes in your diet and lifestyle impact your symptoms over time.

By reviewing this data, you can identify trends, detect areas for improvement, and celebrate successes. It allows you to fine-tune your approach to diverticulitis management, making gradual modifications based on your observations and the guidance of your healthcare professional.

Staying Empowered and Informed

Monitoring symptoms and dietary reactions is not a one-time task but a continuous process. As your body and condition evolve, so too will your dietary needs. By staying attuned to your body, working with healthcare professionals, and making adjustments based on your observations, you are taking an active role in managing your diverticulitis.

Remember to be patient and kind to yourself throughout this journey. Each individual's experience with diverticulitis is unique, and finding the right balance for your body may take time. Embrace the power of personalized nutrition, empower yourself with knowledge, and take pride in your commitment to your health and well-being.

Note: The information provided in this chapter is not intended to replace medical advice. Always consult with your healthcare professional before making any significant changes to your diet or lifestyle.

2.4 Stress and Its Impact on Diverticulitis: Managing More Than Just Your Diet

As you navigate your diverticulitis healing journey, it is essential to recognize the significant role that stress plays in the management of your condition. Stress not only affects your overall well-being but can also impact your diverticulitis symptoms, potentially triggering uncomfortable flare-ups. Therefore, it is crucial to understand the connection between stress and diverticulitis and adopt strategies to effectively manage stress alongside dietary changes.

The Stress-Diverticulitis Connection

Stress is a common part of life for many people, but when it comes to diverticulitis, it can have a direct impact on the health of your gut. When you experience stress, your body releases stress hormones, such as cortisol, which can influence your digestive system.

Stress can lead to a range of responses in the body that may worsen diverticulitis symptoms. One of these responses is a heightened sensitivity in the gut, making it more susceptible to inflammation and irritation. This increased sensitivity may amplify the discomfort caused by diverticulitis and potentially trigger flare-ups.

Furthermore, stress can disrupt the balance of bacteria in your gut. The gut microbiota plays a vital role in maintaining digestive health, and an imbalance can disrupt the normal functioning of the intestines. This imbalance, known as dysbiosis, can contribute to inflammation and further aggravate diverticulitis symptoms.

Coping with Stress: Strategies for Diverticulitis Management

Successfully managing diverticulitis involves more than just dietary adjustments – it requires addressing stress levels as well. By implementing stress management techniques into your routine, you can support your overall well-being and reduce the risk of stress-induced flare-ups. Here are some strategies to consider:

1. Mindfulness and Relaxation Techniques

Practicing mindfulness and relaxation techniques can help you decrease stress levels and promote a sense of calm. Consider incorporating activities such as meditation, deep breathing exercises, and progressive muscle relaxation into your daily routine. These practices can be especially beneficial during times of acute stress or when you notice symptoms of diverticulitis worsening.

2. Regular Physical Activity

Engaging in regular physical activity not only benefits your physical health but also contributes to stress reduction. Exercise releases endorphins, which are natural mood-boosting chemicals, helping to alleviate stress and improve your overall well-being. Choose activities that you enjoy, such as walking, swimming, or yoga, and strive to incorporate them into your routine on a consistent basis.

3. Adequate Sleep

Prioritizing a good night's sleep is essential in managing stress and promoting optimal health. Sleep deprivation can exacerbate stress levels and weaken your immune system, making it more challenging for your body to cope with diverticulitis. Aim for 7-9 hours of quality sleep each night and establish a relaxing bedtime routine to ensure restful sleep.

4. Social Support

Seeking support from loved ones or joining a support group can be invaluable in managing stress associated with diverticulitis. Sharing your experiences, concerns, and triumphs with others who understand can provide emotional relief and a sense of community. Connect with family, friends, or online communities to foster a supportive network that can help you navigate the challenges of living with diverticulitis.

5. Time Management and Prioritization

Efficient time management and setting priorities can reduce stress by creating a sense of control over your daily life. Diverticulitis management often involves making lifestyle adjustments, including dietary changes and self-care practices. Organize your schedule, set realistic goals, and establish healthy boundaries to balance your responsibilities and ensure you have time for stress-reducing activities.

The Importance of a Holistic Approach

While dietary modifications are significant in managing diverticulitis, it is crucial to adopt a holistic approach that encompasses stress management alongside dietary changes. By recognizing the impact of stress on your diverticulitis symptoms and actively implementing stress reduction techniques, you can optimize your overall well-being and enhance the effectiveness of your diverticulitis management plan.

As you incorporate stress management into your routine, remember that everyone's stress triggers and coping mechanisms differ. Explore various strategies and find what works best for you. It may be a combination of techniques or focusing on a single practice that resonates with you personally.

Next Steps: Moving Forward with Confidence

Recognizing the influence of stress on diverticulitis and taking steps to manage it effectively empowers you to actively participate in your own health and well-being. By monitoring your stress levels, adopting stress reduction techniques, and seeking support when needed, you can reduce the risk of stress-induced flare-ups and enhance your diverticulitis management journey.

As you move forward in your healing journey, remember that you are not alone. Reach out to healthcare professionals, support groups, or loved ones for guidance and encouragement. Utilize the resources available to you to ensure you have ample support and reliable information to manage your diverticulitis successfully.

Chapter 3: Dietary Foundations for Diverticulitis

3.1 Safe Foods: Building Your Diverticulitis-Friendly Pantry

When it comes to managing diverticulitis through diet, one of the most critical steps you can take is to build a diverticulitis-friendly pantry. By stocking your kitchen with safe, nutritious ingredients, you can reduce the risk of triggering painful flare-ups and ensure you have a variety of options for preparing delicious, nourishing meals.

Diverticulitis and Safe Foods

When you have diverticulitis, the focus of your diet should be on foods that are easy to digest and low in fiber. These foods can help reduce inflammation and irritation in your digestive tract, making it easier for your body to heal.

Some of the most recommended diverticulitis-safe foods include:

- Lean protein sources like chicken, fish, turkey, and eggs
- Low-fiber fruits like cantaloupe, bananas, and honeydew melon
- Cooked or canned vegetables like carrots, green beans, and beets
- Low-fiber grains like white rice, pasta, and refined bread
- Fermented foods like yogurt and kefir

On the other hand, certain foods can aggravate diverticulitis symptoms and must be avoided. These include:

- High-fiber foods like whole grains, beans, legumes, fruits with skin, and vegetables with seeds and skin
- Nuts and seeds
- Spicy foods
- Caffeine and alcohol

By understanding which foods are safe to eat and which should be avoided, you can build a diverticulitis-friendly pantry that promotes optimal digestive health.

Stocking Your Pantry with Safe Foods

Here are some ingredients that can be included in your pantry to help support your diverticulitis management:

1. Low-Fiber Grains

Low-fiber grains, such as white rice, pasta, and refined bread, can be used as the foundation of many diverticulitis-safe dishes. These ingredients are easy to digest and can be cooked in a variety of ways, making them incredibly versatile.

2. Lean Proteins

Lean proteins like chicken, turkey, fish, and eggs are essential for providing your body with energy and essential nutrients. They are easy to digest and can be cooked in various ways, making them a staple in any diverticulitis-friendly pantry.

3. Low-Fiber Fruits and Vegetables

Low-fiber fruits and vegetables are critical for providing your body with essential nutrients while keeping your digestive system healthy. Canned or cooked vegetables like carrots, beets, and green beans, and low-fiber fruits like cantaloupe, bananas, and honeydew melon, are safe choices to include in your pantry.

4. Fermented Foods

Fermented foods like yogurt and kefir can be beneficial for promoting a healthy gut microbiome. These foods contain probiotics that can help maintain a balanced bacterial environment in your gut, reducing the risk of inflammation and irritation. Be sure to choose unsweetened and unflavored options.

5. Spices and Seasonings

While spicy foods can exacerbate diverticulitis symptoms, mild spices like oregano, basil, and thyme can be used to add flavor to your meals without causing discomfort. Additionally, salt-free seasonings like garlic powder, onion powder, and lemon juice can be used to enhance the taste of your dishes without aggravating your condition.

In addition to these essentials, consider incorporating broth, canned fruits and vegetables, nut butters (without added seeds), and pureed fruits and vegetables into your pantry. These ingredients can be used in a variety of dishes and can provide your body with the essential nutrients it needs to support your overall health.

Creating Diverticulitis-Friendly Meals

Once you have built your pantry, you can begin creating meals that are safe, nutritious, and delicious.

By incorporating diverticulitis-safe ingredients into your meals and choosing recipes that are easy to digest, you can reduce the risk of triggering painful symptoms while promoting optimal health.

Building a diverticulitis-friendly pantry is an essential step in managing your condition through diet. By stocking your kitchen with low-fiber grains, lean proteins, low-fiber fruits and vegetables, fermented foods, and mild spices, you can create meals that are both delicious and safe for your digestive system.

3.2 Foods to Avoid: Understanding Potential Triggers

The management of diverticulitis through diet is crucial for reducing the risk of painful flare-ups and promoting overall digestive health. While building a diverticulitis-friendly pantry is an essential step, it is equally important to understand which foods to avoid. Certain foods can trigger inflammation and discomfort in the digestive system, causing symptoms to worsen. By recognizing and eliminating these potential triggers, you can regain control over your health and minimize the impact of diverticulitis on your daily life.

The Problematic Culprits: Foods to Stay Away From

To effectively manage diverticulitis, it is essential to be aware of the foods that can potentially aggravate your condition. While the specifics may vary from person to person, the following categories of foods are commonly associated with triggering symptoms. It's important to note that the effects of these foods might differ based on individual sensitivity and the stage of your condition.

1. High-Fiber Foods

High-fiber foods are generally recommended for maintaining a healthy digestive system. However, when it comes to diverticulitis, these same foods can exacerbate symptoms by placing additional strain on the inflamed areas of the colon. Foods to avoid in this category include:

- **Whole grains:** Products such as whole wheat bread, whole grain pasta, and brown rice should be avoided due to their high fiber content.
- **Legumes and beans:** Foods like lentils, chickpeas, kidney beans, and black beans are rich sources of fiber and can be difficult to digest, leading to increased discomfort.
- **Fruits and vegetables with skin**: While fruits and vegetables are typically good for overall health, the skin of certain varieties can be tough to digest. Avoid fruits like apples and pears, as well as vegetables like broccoli and Brussels sprouts, which can contain irritating fibers.

2. Nuts and Seeds

Nuts and seeds are known for their high fiber and fat content. Although they provide many health benefits, they can also irritate the diverticula and worsen symptoms. **Examples of nuts and seeds to avoid include:**

- Almonds
- Walnuts

- Chia seeds
- Flaxseeds
- Sesame seeds
- Sunflower seeds

3. Spicy Foods

For individuals living with diverticulitis, spicy foods can be especially problematic. These foods can irritate the digestive tract, potentially leading to inflammation and discomfort. Common spicy ingredients to steer clear of include:

- Chili peppers
- Cayenne pepper
- Hot sauces
- Peppercorns

4. Caffeine and Alcohol

Both caffeine and alcohol can have negative effects on the digestive system and may cause symptoms to worsen. It's advisable to limit or avoid these substances to manage diverticulitis effectively. Examples of beverages to limit or avoid include:

- Coffee
- Tea
- Carbonated drinks
- Alcoholic beverages

While it may seem challenging to avoid these foods entirely, especially if they have been staples in your diet, making gradual changes and exploring alternative options can significantly benefit your digestive health.

Navigating the Elimination Process: A Step-by-Step Approach

Understanding which foods to eliminate is just the beginning. Experimenting with your diet and identifying specific triggers can help you personalize your approach to managing diverticulitis. It is recommended to follow a step-by-step process to determine which foods are tolerable for your unique situation. Here's a suggested approach:

1. Keep a Food Diary

Start by keeping a detailed food diary, noting everything you consume and any symptoms experienced afterward. This record can help identify patterns and potential trigger foods.

2. Gradually Eliminate Certain Foods

Based on your food diary, gradually eliminate potential trigger foods one at a time. This can help determine which specific items are causing or exacerbating symptoms. Eliminate each food for a week or two to allow sufficient time for your body to react and for symptoms to subside.

3. Monitor Symptoms

During the elimination process, closely monitor your symptoms. Are they improving or remaining relatively stable? If they continue to persist or worsen, it's possible that other foods or factors not yet identified may be contributing to your discomfort.

4. Reintroduce Foods

After eliminating specific foods and experiencing relief from symptoms, gradually reintroduce them back into your diet, one at a time. Take note of any changes in symptoms or the return of discomfort. This can help identify specific trigger foods that should be avoided in the long term.

5. Seek Professional Guidance

If you find the elimination process challenging or you're unsure about which foods to eliminate or reintroduce, consider seeking guidance from a registered dietitian or healthcare professional who specializes in digestive health. They can provide personalized recommendations based on your needs and guide you through the process effectively.

By adopting a systematic approach to identify trigger foods, you can establish a clear understanding of what works best for your body. This knowledge empowers you to make informed choices and regain control over your diverticulitis management.

Avoiding potential trigger foods is an integral part of effectively managing diverticulitis through diet. By understanding which foods to stay away from and following a step-by-step approach to identify your personal triggers, you can reduce the risk of triggering painful symptoms and gain control over your digestive health. While it may require adjustments to your eating habits, the long-term benefits of a well-managed diet are well worth the effort. Remember, it's important to consult a healthcare professional for personalized guidance to ensure you are making the right choices for your unique situation.

3.3 The Importance of Hydration: Best Practices for Fluid Intake

When it comes to managing diverticulitis, the role of hydration in supporting digestive health cannot be overstated. Adequate fluid intake is crucial for maintaining regularity, preventing constipation, and minimizing the risk of painful flare-ups. As you navigate through your diverticulitis management journey, understanding the significance of hydration and implementing best practices for fluid intake can empower you to take proactive steps toward improving your overall well-being. This section will provide you with valuable insights on the importance of hydration and practical recommendations for optimizing your fluid intake, catering to individuals like yourself who seek reliable and clear guidance on managing diverticulitis through diet.

The Role of Hydration in Digestive Health

Before delving into specific hydration recommendations, it's essential to comprehend the critical role that adequate fluid intake plays in supporting digestive health, particularly for individuals managing diverticulitis. Hydration is fundamental for the following reasons:

1. Preventing Constipation

In the context of diverticulitis, maintaining regular bowel movements is vital for minimizing strain on the digestive system and reducing the risk of complications. Adequate hydration helps soften stools, making them easier to pass and reducing the likelihood of constipation, a common issue associated with diverticulitis.

2. Supporting Digestive Function

Hydration is essential for aiding the body's digestive processes, including the breakdown and absorption of nutrients from food. By ensuring optimal fluid intake, you can support the efficient functioning of your digestive system, potentially reducing discomfort and symptoms associated with diverticulitis.

3. Minimizing the Risk of Flare-Ups

Well-regulated hydration can play a significant role in minimizing the risk of painful diverticulitis flare-ups. Proper hydration helps maintain a healthy balance within your digestive tract, reducing the likelihood of inflammation and discomfort associated with the condition.

Practical Recommendations for Optimizing Fluid Intake

Now that we recognize the pivotal role of hydration in managing diverticulitis, incorporating practical strategies for optimizing fluid intake becomes essential. Below are several actionable recommendations tailored to your needs, aiming to provide you with clear and reliable guidance on how to maximize the benefits of proper hydration:

1. Water: The Foundation of Hydration

Water serves as the cornerstone of effective hydration. It is recommended to consume at least eight 8-ounce glasses of water per day to maintain adequate fluid levels in the body. To enhance hydration, consider infusing your water with slices of refreshing citrus fruits or opting for herbal teas, contributing additional flavor while promoting increased fluid intake.

2. Hydrating Foods

In addition to consuming liquids, incorporating hydrating foods into your diet can contribute to your overall fluid intake. Examples of hydrating foods include cucumber, watermelon, strawberries, and lettuce. These foods are not only rich in essential nutrients but also aid in maintaining hydration levels within the body.

3. Limiting Dehydrating Substances

Certain beverages and substances can lead to dehydration and should be consumed in moderation or avoided. Caffeinated drinks and alcohol are known to have diuretic effects, contributing to increased fluid loss. While it may not be necessary to eliminate these entirely, it is advisable to limit their consumption and balance them with increased water intake to mitigate their dehydrating effects.

4. Monitoring Urine Color

A simple and effective way to gauge your hydration levels is to monitor the color of your urine. Clear to light yellow urine indicates well-hydrated status, while darker yellow urine may signify dehydration. By paying attention to this visual indicator, you can adjust your fluid intake as needed to maintain optimal hydration levels.

5. Consistency and Awareness

Establishing a consistent pattern of fluid intake throughout the day is essential for maintaining proper hydration. Rather than consuming large quantities of fluids at once, aim for regular, evenly spaced intervals to support your body's hydration needs. Additionally, raising awareness of your hydration habits and emphasizing the importance of fluid intake in your daily routine can help cultivate a proactive approach to managing diverticulitis.

Empowering Your Hydration Journey

In conclusion, prioritizing hydration as a fundamental aspect of diverticulitis management through diet is an empowering endeavor. By recognizing the various benefits of adequate fluid intake and integrating practical strategies into your daily routine, you are taking vital steps toward enhancing your digestive health and minimizing the impact of diverticulitis on your overall well-being. As you embark on this journey, remember that the recommended strategies are designed to provide you with accessible, reliable, and clear guidance, ensuring that you can confidently navigate the complexities of managing diverticulitis through optimal hydration practices. By incorporating these recommendations into your daily routine, you will undoubtedly cultivate a balanced, enjoyable diet that promotes digestive health and empowers you to take charge of your well-being.

Remember, by being attentive to your body's hydration needs and adopting practical strategies, you are not only managing your diverticulitis effectively but also enhancing your overall quality of life.

3.4 Balancing Nutrients: Proteins, Fats, and Carbohydrates

When it comes to managing diverticulitis through diet, achieving a balanced intake of nutrients is crucial for supporting your overall health and well-being. A well-rounded diet should include a careful balance of proteins, fats, and carbohydrates to provide the necessary fuel and building blocks your body needs. In this section, we will explore the significance of each macronutrient and provide practical guidance on how to strike the right balance for optimal nutrition while managing diverticulitis.

Proteins: Building Blocks for Health

Proteins are essential for the growth, repair, and maintenance of tissues within your body. They are made up of amino acids which play vital roles in various bodily functions. Incorporating sufficient protein into your diet is essential for managing diverticulitis and supporting the healing process. High-quality sources of protein include lean meats, poultry, fish, eggs, dairy products, legumes, and plant-based alternatives such as tofu and tempeh.

When selecting protein sources, opt for lean cuts of meat and trim off any visible fat. For those following vegetarian or vegan diets, legumes such as lentils, chickpeas, and beans are excellent sources of protein. Including a variety of protein sources in your meals ensures you receive a wide range of essential amino acids, promoting good health and supporting your body's healing processes.

Fats: The Right Choices for Optimal Health

While fats have often been criticized, it's important to note that not all fats are created equal. Incorporating healthy fats into your diet is crucial for managing diverticulitis and supporting your overall well-being. Healthy fats provide energy, support cell growth, protect organs, and help absorb certain vitamins.

Include monounsaturated and polyunsaturated fats in your diet by incorporating foods such as avocados, olive oil, nuts, and seeds. These healthy fats can help reduce inflammation and promote heart health. It's important to limit saturated and trans fats, which can increase inflammation and raise the risk of heart disease. Minimize your intake of foods like butter, full-fat dairy products, and fatty cuts of meat.

Carbohydrates: Fuel for Energy

Carbohydrates are the body's primary source of energy, making them an essential component of your diet. However, not all carbohydrates are equal. Opt for complex carbohydrates, which are rich in fiber, as they provide sustained energy and support digestive health. Whole grains, legumes, fruits, and vegetables are excellent sources of complex carbohydrates.

When managing diverticulitis, it's important to pay attention to the fiber content of carbohydrates. Gradually increase your fiber intake to promote regular bowel movements and prevent constipation. However, it's essential to strike a balance, as excessive amounts of fiber can lead to discomfort or gas. Seek guidance from a registered dietitian or healthcare professional to determine the appropriate fiber intake for your specific needs.

Striking the Balance: Practical Tips

To strike the right balance of macronutrients while managing diverticulitis, consider the following practical tips:

Portion Control: Pay attention to portion sizes, as consuming excessive amounts of any macronutrient can be detrimental to your health. Use measuring tools to ensure accurate portion sizes and consider working with a registered dietitian who can provide personalized guidance on portion control.

Meal Planning: Plan your meals in advance to ensure a balanced distribution of macronutrients throughout the day. Include a source of lean protein, healthy fats, and complex carbohydrates in each meal to promote satiety and sustained energy.

Adequate Hydration: Don't forget the importance of staying hydrated while balancing your macronutrients. Proper hydration supports digestion and helps prevent constipation, ensuring your body can effectively utilize the nutrients you consume.

Individualization: Each person's dietary needs and tolerances may vary. If you find certain foods trigger uncomfortable symptoms or flare-ups, consider working with a healthcare professional or registered dietitian to customize your diet and identify any specific sensitivities.

Practical Examples

To provide you with some practical examples of balanced meals, consider these options:

- Grilled chicken breast (protein) accompanied by a salad with mixed greens and a drizzle of olive oil (healthy fat), and a side of quinoa (complex carbohydrate).
- Baked salmon (protein) served with sautéed vegetables cooked in a small amount of avocado oil (healthy fat), and a serving of sweet potatoes (complex carbohydrate).
- Vegetable stir-fry with tofu (protein), cooked with a sprinkle of sesame oil (healthy fat), and served over a bed of brown rice (complex carbohydrate).

Remember, these examples are meant to illustrate the principles of balanced nutrition. It's essential to personalize your diet based on personal preferences, dietary restrictions, and stage of diverticulitis. Consulting with a registered dietitian can provide valuable insights and guidance in developing a customized meal plan that meets your needs.

Achieving a balance of proteins, fats, and carbohydrates is essential for managing diverticulitis through diet. Understanding the importance of each macronutrient and making informed choices helps support your overall health and reduces the risk of triggering uncomfortable symptoms or flare-ups. Remember to focus on high-quality protein sources, choose healthy fats, and incorporate complex carbohydrates into your meals. With proper portion control, meal planning, and individualization of your diet, you can enjoy a balanced and enjoyable eating experience while effectively managing your diverticulitis.

Chapter 4: Recipes for Relief and Recovery

4.1 Breakfast Recipes: A Gentle Start to Your Day

Starting your morning with a nourishing breakfast sets the tone for a day of healing and well-being when managing diverticulitis. Enjoying a gentle and balanced meal to kick off your day can provide essential nutrients and energy without triggering digestive discomfort. In this section, we will explore practical and delicious breakfast recipes designed to support your digestive health and help you feel your best.

Nourishing Morning Meals

Breakfast is often referred to as the most important meal of the day, and this sentiment holds true when managing diverticulitis. A nourishing breakfast can help stabilize blood sugar levels, kickstart your metabolism, and provide your body with essential nutrients to support digestion and overall health. By incorporating the right ingredients and balance of nutrients into your morning meal, you can set yourself up for a day of wellness and vitality.

Guidelines for Digestive-Friendly Breakfasts

When planning your breakfast meals, it's important to consider the following guidelines to ensure they are gentle on your digestive system:

Opt for Fiber-Rich Options: Choose breakfast foods that are rich in fiber, such as whole grains, fruits, and vegetables. Fiber helps promote healthy digestion, regulate bowel movements, and support gut health. Oatmeal topped with berries, chia seeds, and a dollop of Greek yogurt is a fiber-rich and satisfying breakfast option that can be gentle on your digestive system.

Include Protein Sources: Incorporating protein into your breakfast is essential for muscle repair and energy. Choose lean protein sources like eggs, Greek yogurt, or nut butter to provide sustained energy throughout the morning. A vegetable omelet made with spinach, tomatoes, and feta cheese is a protein-packed breakfast that can keep you feeling full and satisfied.

Embrace Healthy Fats: Including healthy fats in your breakfast can help promote satiety and aid in the absorption of fat-soluble vitamins. Avocado, nuts, seeds, and olive oil are excellent sources of healthy fats that can be easily incorporated into your morning meal. Try spreading avocado on whole grain toast and topping it with sliced tomatoes and a sprinkle of sea salt for a nutritious and delicious breakfast option.

4.1.1 Smoothies and Juices: Nutrient-Dense Morning Boosters

Recipe 1: Berry Green Smoothie

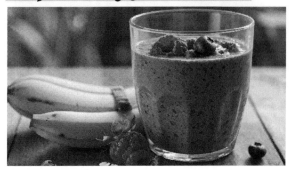

Preparation time = 5 minutes

Ingredients =

- 1 cup of spinach
- 1/2 cup of mixed berries (such as strawberries, blueberries, and raspberries)
- 1/2 banana
- 1 cup of almond milk
- 1 tablespoon of chia seeds

Servings = Serves 1

Mode of cooking: Blending

Procedure:

Add all of the ingredients to a blender and blend until smooth. Serve immediately.

Nutritional values: 250 calories | 7g protein | 8g fat | 40g carbohydrates

Recipe 2: Tropical Turmeric Smoothie

Preparation time = 5 minutes

Ingredients =

- 1/2 cup of pineapple chunks
- 1/2 cup of mango chunks
- 1/2 banana
- 1 cup of coconut water
- 1/2 teaspoon of turmeric powder

Servings = Serves 1

Mode of cooking: Blending

Procedure:

Add all of the ingredients to a blender and blend until smooth. Serve immediately.

Nutritional values: 220 calories | 2g protein | 1g fat | 53g carbohydrates

Recipe 3: Cucumber and Mint Juice

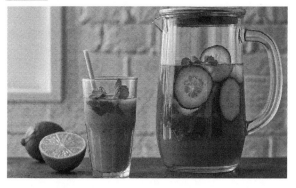

Preparation time = 10 minutes

Ingredients =

- 1 cucumber
- Handful of fresh mint leaves
- Juice of 1 lime
- 1 cup of water

Servings = Serves 1

Mode of cooking: Blending

Procedure:

Peel and chop the cucumber. Add the cucumber, mint leaves, lime juice, and water to a blender. Blend until smooth. Strain the juice through a fine-mesh sieve to remove any pulp. Serve chilled.

Nutritional values: 40 calories | 1g protein | 0g fat | 10g carbohydrates

Recipe 4: Carrot and Ginger Smoothie

Preparation time = 5 minutes

Ingredients =

- 1 large carrot, peeled and chopped
- 1/2 inch piece of fresh ginger, grated
- 1/2 banana
- 1 cup of almond milk
- 1 tablespoon of honey (optional)

Servings = Serves 1

Mode of cooking: Blending

Procedure:

Add all of the ingredients to a blender and blend until smooth. Add honey if desired for added sweetness. Serve immediately.

Nutritional values: 200 calories | 4g protein | 4g fat | 39g carbohydrates

Recipe 5: Spinach and Apple Juice

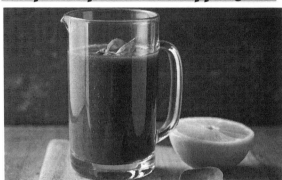

Preparation time = 10 minutes

Ingredients =

- 2 cups of fresh spinach
- 1 apple, cored and chopped
- Juice of 1 lemon
- 1 cup of water

Servings = Serves 1

Mode of cooking: Blending

Procedure:

Add all of the ingredients to a blender and blend until smooth. Strain the juice through a fine-mesh sieve to remove any pulp. Serve chilled.

Nutritional values: 70 calories | 2g protein | 0g fat | 18g carbohydrates

4.1.2 Porridge and Warm Cereals: Soothing Whole Grain Options

Recipe 1: Quinoa Porridge

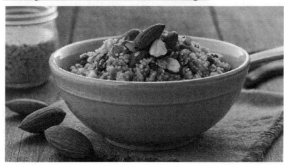

Preparation time = 15 minutes

Ingredients =

- 1/2 cup of quinoa
- 1 cup of almond milk
- 1/2 teaspoon of cinnamon
- 1 tablespoon of honey or maple syrup
- Fresh fruits and nuts for topping (optional)

Servings = Serves 2

Mode of cooking: Stovetop

Procedure:

Rinse quinoa under cold water. In a saucepan, bring almond milk and quinoa to a boil.

Reduce heat, cover, and simmer for 10-15 minutes until the quinoa is cooked and the mixture has thickened. Stir in cinnamon and sweetener of choice. Serve hot with fresh fruits and nuts as desired.

Nutritional values: 310 calories | 9g protein | 8g fat | 52g carbohydrates

Recipe 2: Brown Rice Pudding

Preparation time = 10 minutes

Ingredients =

- 1 cup of cooked brown rice
- 1 cup of almond milk
- 1 tablespoon of honey or maple syrup
- 1/4 teaspoon of vanilla extract
- Cinnamon for garnish

Servings = Serves 2

Mode of cooking: Stovetop

Procedure:

In a saucepan, combine cooked brown rice, almond milk, honey or maple syrup, and vanilla extract. Heat the mixture over medium heat, stirring occasionally, until it reaches a simmer. Reduce heat to low and continue to cook for about 5 minutes until the mixture thickens. Remove from heat and let it cool slightly. Serve warm, sprinkled with cinnamon.

Nutritional values: 282 calories | 5g protein | 4g fat | 56g carbohydrates

Recipe 3: Buckwheat Porridge

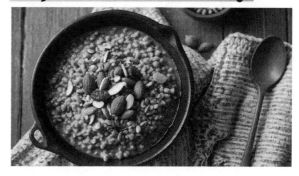

Preparation time = 20 minutes

Ingredients =

- 1/2 cup of buckwheat groats

- 1 cup of almond milk
- 1/2 teaspoon of cinnamon
- 1 tablespoon of honey or maple syrup
- Fresh fruits and nuts for topping (optional)

Servings = Serves 2

Mode of cooking: Stovetop

Procedure:

Rinse buckwheat groats under cold water. In a saucepan, bring almond milk and buckwheat groats to a boil. Reduce heat, cover, and simmer for 15-20 minutes until the buckwheat is cooked and the mixture has thickened. Stir in cinnamon and sweetener of choice. Serve hot with fresh fruits and nuts as desired.

Nutritional values: 320 calories | 11g protein | 5g fat | 61g carbohydrates

Recipe 4: Oatmeal with Apples and Cinnamon

Preparation time = 10 minutes

Ingredients =

- 1 cup of rolled oats
- 1 cup of water
- 1 cup of almond milk
- 1 apple, peeled and chopped
- 1/2 teaspoon of cinnamon
- 1 tablespoon of honey or maple syrup (optional)

Servings = Serves 2

Mode of cooking: Stovetop

Procedure:

In a saucepan, bring water, almond milk, and rolled oats to a boil.

Reduce heat and simmer for about 5 minutes, stirring occasionally. Add the chopped apple and cinnamon to the mixture and continue to cook for another 5 minutes or until the oats have reached the desired consistency. Stir in honey or maple syrup if desired. Serve hot.

Nutritional values: 275 calories | 7g protein | 4g fat | 52g carbohydrates

Recipe 5: Millet Porridge with Berries

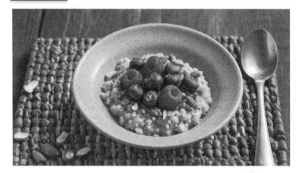

Preparation time = 15 minutes

Ingredients =

- 1/2 cup of millet
- 1 cup of almond milk
- 1 cup of water
- 1 tablespoon of honey or maple syrup
- 1/2 cup of mixed berries
- Chopped nuts for topping (optional)

Servings = Serves 2

Mode of cooking: Stovetop

Procedure:

Rinse millet under cold water. In a saucepan, combine millet, almond milk, and water. Bring to a boil.

Reduce heat, cover, and simmer for 10-15 minutes until the millet is cooked and the mixture has thickened. Stir in honey or maple syrup. Serve hot, topped with mixed berries and chopped nuts if desired.

Nutritional values: 285 calories | 5g protein | 5g fat | 55g carbohydrates

4.1.3 Egg Dishes: Protein-Rich Breakfasts with a Gentle Touch

Recipe 1: Scrambled Eggs with Spinach

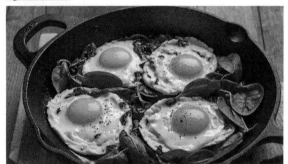

Preparation time = 10 minutes

Ingredients

- 2 eggs
- 1 cup of fresh spinach
- Salt and pepper to taste

Servings = Serves 1

Mode of cooking: Stovetop

Procedure:

In a non-stick skillet, heat a little oil or cooking spray over medium heat. Beat the eggs in a bowl and season with salt and pepper. Add the spinach to the skillet and sauté until wilted. Pour the beaten eggs into the skillet and scramble them gently until cooked to your desired level of doneness.

Serve hot.

Nutritional values: Approximately 230 calories | 18g protein | 16g fat | 3g carbohydrates

Recipe 2: Baked Eggs with Vegetables

Preparation time = 20 minutes

Ingredients

- 2 eggs
- 1/2 cup of chopped bell peppers
- 1/4 cup of diced tomatoes
- Salt and pepper to taste

Servings = Serves 1

Mode of cooking: Oven

Procedure:

Preheat your oven to 350°F (175°C). Grease a small oven-safe dish with oil or cooking spray. In the dish, combine the chopped bell peppers, diced tomatoes, salt, and pepper. Carefully crack the eggs on top of the vegetable mixture. Bake in the preheated oven for about

12-15 minutes until the eggs are cooked to your desired level of doneness. Serve hot.

Nutritional values: Approximately 180 calories | 12g protein | 12g fat | 4g carbohydrates

---

Recipe 3: Poached Eggs with Asparagus

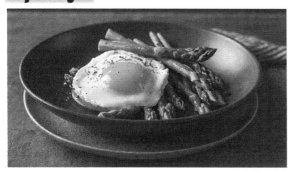

Preparation time = 15 minutes

Ingredients

- eggs
- 1 cup of asparagus spears
- Salt and pepper to taste2

Servings = Serves 1

Mode of cooking: Stovetop

Procedure:

Fill a saucepan with water and bring it to a gentle boil. Meanwhile, wash and trim the asparagus spears. Add the asparagus to the boiling water and cook for about 2-3 minutes until tender-crisp. Remove the asparagus from the water with tongs and set aside. Reduce the heat, creating a gentle simmer in the saucepan. Crack the eggs into separate small bowls or ramekins. Carefully slide each egg into the simmering water.

Poach the eggs for about 3-4 minutes until the whites are set and the yolks are still runny. Remove the poached eggs from the water using a slotted spoon. Serve the poached eggs over the cooked asparagus, seasoned with salt and pepper.

Nutritional values: Approximately 180 calories | 12g protein | 12g fat | 2g carbohydrates

---

Recipe 4: Vegetable Omelet

Preparation time = 15 minutes

Ingredients

- 2 eggs
- 1/4 cup of diced bell peppers
- 1/4 cup of diced zucchini
- 1/4 cup of diced mushrooms |
- Salt and pepper to taste

Servings = Serves 1

Mode of cooking: Stovetop

Procedure:

In a non-stick skillet, heat a little oil or cooking spray over medium heat. Add the diced bell peppers, zucchini, and mushrooms to the skillet and sauté until they are slightly softened.

In a bowl, beat the eggs and season with salt and pepper. Pour the beaten eggs over the sautéed vegetables in the skillet. Cook the omelet, occasionally lifting the edges with a spatula to allow the uncooked eggs to flow underneath. Continue cooking until the omelet is set, but still slightly runny on top. Fold the omelet in half and cook for another minute until fully set. Serve hot.

Nutritional values: Approximately 230 calories | 18g protein | 16g fat | 5g carbohydrates

Recipe 5: Egg and Avocado Salad

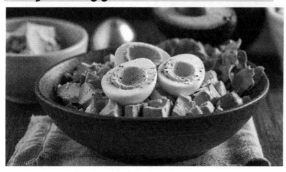

Preparation time = 10 minutes

- **Ingredients** 2 boiled eggs, peeled and chopped
- 1 small avocado, peeled and diced
- 1 tablespoon of lemon juice |
- Salt and pepper to taste

Servings = Serves 1

Mode of cooking: None (Eggs are boiled)

Procedure:

In a bowl, combine the chopped boiled eggs and diced avocado. Drizzle lemon juice over the mixture and gently toss to coat. Season with salt and pepper to taste.

Serve as a salad or enjoy it on whole-grain toast.

Nutritional values: Approximately 280 calories | 14g protein | 24g fat | 8g carbohydrates

4.1.4 Breakfast Breads and Pastries: Fiber-Enriched Bites for the Morning

Recipe 1: Oat Bran Muffins

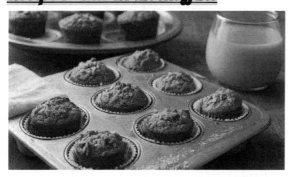

Preparation time = 30 minutes

Ingredients

- 1 cup oat bran
- 1/2 cup whole wheat flour
- 1/4 cup unsweetened applesauce
- 1/4 cup honey
- 1 tsp baking powder

Servings = Makes 6 muffins

Mode of cooking: Oven

Procedure:

Preheat the oven to 375°F (190°C) and line a muffin pan with liners. In a bowl, mix oat bran, whole wheat flour, baking powder, applesauce, and honey until well combined. Divide the batter among the muffin cups. Bake for 15-18 minutes or until a toothpick inserted comes out clean. Allow the muffins to cool before serving.

Nutritional values: Approximately 120 calories | 4g protein | 2g fat | 24g carbohydrates

Recipe 2: Flaxseed Banana Bread

Preparation time = 50 minutes

Ingredients

- 1 cup ground flaxseed
- 2 ripe bananas, mashed
- 2 eggs
- 1/4 cup honey
- 1 tsp baking soda

Servings = Makes 1 loaf

Mode of cooking: Oven

Procedure:

Preheat the oven to 350°F (175°C) and grease a loaf pan. In a bowl, mix ground flaxseed, mashed bananas, eggs, honey, and baking soda until well combined. Pour the batter into the prepared loaf pan. Bake for 35-40 minutes or until a toothpick inserted comes out clean. Allow the banana bread to cool before slicing and serving.

Nutritional values: Approximately 150 calories | 5g protein | 8g fat | 15g carbohydrates

Recipe 3: Chia Seed Breakfast Bars

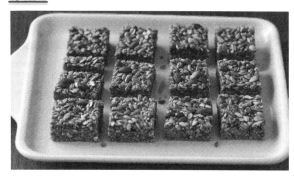

Preparation time = 40 minutes

Ingredients

- 1/2 cup chia seeds
- 1/4 cup almond butter
- 1/4 cup maple syrup
- 1/4 cup chopped nuts

Servings = Makes 8 bars

Mode of cooking: Refrigeration

Procedure:

In a bowl, mix chia seeds, almond butter, and maple syrup until well combined. Stir in chopped nuts. Press the mixture into a lined baking pan and refrigerate for at least 30 minutes. Cut into bars before serving.

Nutritional values: Approximately 180 calories | 5g protein | 10g fat | 15g carbohydrates

Recipe 4: Quinoa Breakfast Cookies

Preparation time = 40 minutes

Ingredients

- 1 cup cooked quinoa
- 1/4 cup almond butter
- 1/4 cup dried cranberries
- | 1 tsp cinnamon

Servings = Makes 12 cookies

Mode of cooking: Oven

Procedure:

Preheat the oven to 350°F (175°C) and line a baking sheet with parchment paper. In a bowl, mix cooked quinoa, almond butter, dried cranberries, and cinnamon until well combined. Scoop spoonfuls of the mixture onto the prepared baking sheet and flatten slightly. Bake for 20-25 minutes or until the cookies are set. Allow the cookies to cool before serving.

Nutritional values: Approximately 100 calories | 3g protein | 5g fat | 15g carbohydrates

Recipe 5: Sweet Potato Breakfast Bars

Preparation time = 45 minutes

Ingredients

- 1 cup mashed sweet potato
- 1/2 cup rolled oats
- 1/4 cup chopped walnuts
- 1/4 cup raisins

Servings = Makes 6 bars

Mode of cooking: Oven

Procedure:

Preheat the oven to 375°F (190°C) and grease a baking dish. In a bowl, mix mashed sweet potato, rolled oats, chopped walnuts, and raisins until well combined. Press the mixture into the prepared baking dish. Bake for 25-30 minutes or until the bars are firm. Allow the bars to cool before cutting into squares.

Nutritional values: Approximately 130 calories | 3g protein | 5g fat | 20g carbohydrates

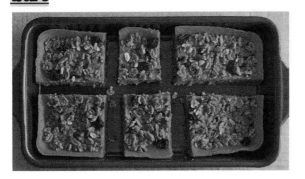

4.2 Nourishing Lunches: Meals That Fuel and Heal

These fiber-enriched breakfast bread and pastry recipes are nutritious and suitable for individuals following a diverticulitis diet.

Incorporating a nourishing lunch into your daily routine is essential for managing diverticulitis and promoting overall digestive health. Choosing the right ingredients and preparing balanced meals can help fuel your body while providing the necessary nutrients to support healing. In this section, we will explore practical and tasty lunch ideas that will keep you satisfied and contribute to your well-being.

Understanding the Importance of Nourishment

Lunchtime presents an opportunity to refuel your body and replenish energy levels. When managing diverticulitis, it is crucial to prioritize meals that nourish your digestive system and provide the nutrients your body needs. A balanced lunch can provide a combination of fiber, protein, healthy fats, vitamins, and minerals to support gut health and reduce the risk of triggering painful flare-ups.

Guidelines for Nourishing Lunches

When planning your lunch meals, consider the following guidelines to create nourishing options:

Focus on Fiber-Rich Foods: Include fiber-rich foods in your lunch as they promote regular bowel movements and prevent constipation. Opt for whole grains, such as quinoa, brown rice, or whole-wheat pasta, as the base for your lunch meals. Add in a variety of fruits and vegetables, like leafy greens, bell peppers, broccoli, and berries, to increase the fiber content and provide valuable vitamins and antioxidants.

Incorporate Lean Protein: Include lean sources of protein in your lunch to support muscle health and aid in the healing process. Opt for skinless poultry, fish, tofu, or legumes like beans or lentils. These protein sources are easier to digest and less likely to irritate the digestive system compared to fatty cuts of meat or processed meats.

Choose Healthy Fats: Incorporate healthy fats into your lunch, such as avocado, nuts, seeds, or olive oil. Healthy fats are important for nutrient absorption, satiety, and overall health. They also support a balanced inflammatory response, which is beneficial for managing diverticulitis.

Avoid Trigger Foods: Be cautious of foods that can potentially trigger symptoms or flare-ups. While trigger foods may vary from person to person, common ones include spicy foods, high-fat foods, processed foods, and foods with added sugars. It's best to avoid these foods during lunchtime to minimize the risk of discomfort or inflammation.

Nourishing Lunch Ideas

To help you incorporate these guidelines into practical lunch meals, here are a few nourishing lunch ideas:

Quinoa Salad with Roasted Vegetables: Prepare a colorful salad by mixing cooked quinoa with an assortment of roasted vegetables like cherry tomatoes, zucchini, bell peppers, and red onions. Toss with a light vinaigrette made from olive oil, lemon juice, and your choice of herbs. Add some grilled chicken breast or chickpeas for added protein.

Lentil and Vegetable Soup: Create a hearty and filling soup by simmering lentils, carrots, celery, and spinach in a flavorful vegetable broth. Season with herbs and spices such as thyme, bay leaves, and cumin. Pair with a side of whole grain bread or crackers for a satisfying lunch.

Grilled Salmon with Steamed Veggies: Grill a fresh salmon filet and serve it alongside a medley of steamed vegetables like broccoli, cauliflower, and carrots. Drizzle with a lemon-dill sauce and accompany with a side of quinoa or brown rice for a well-rounded meal.

Veggie Wrap with Hummus: Fill a whole wheat tortilla with an array of colorful vegetables such as spinach, cucumber, bell peppers, and grated carrots. Spread a generous layer of hummus for added flavor and plant-based protein. Roll it up and enjoy a convenient, nutrient-packed lunch.

Nourishing lunches play a significant role in managing diverticulitis and supporting digestive health. By following the guidelines provided, you can create balanced and delicious lunch options that contribute to your overall well-being. Focus on incorporating fiber-rich foods, lean proteins, and healthy fats, while avoiding trigger foods that may aggravate your symptoms. With these ideas and a little creativity, you can enjoy nourishing lunches that not only provide essential nutrients but also help you maintain control of your diverticulitis management journey.

Salads: Colorful, Fiber-Filled Combinations

Salads are a delightful way to incorporate a wide array of nutrients into your meals while managing diverticulitis. Packed with fiber and bursting with flavor, these colorful combinations will not only satiate your taste buds but also nourish your body. In this section, we will explore five nourishing salad recipes that are ideal for a diverticulitis-friendly diet.

4.2.1 Salads: Colorful, Fiber-Filled Combinations

Recipe 1: Mediterranean Chickpea Salad

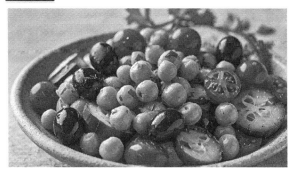

Preparation time: 15 minutes

Ingredients:

- 1 can (15 oz) chickpeas, rinsed and drained
- 1 cup cherry tomatoes, halved
- 1 cucumber, diced
- 1/2 red onion, thinly sliced
- 1/4 cup Kalamata olives, pitted and halved
- 2 tbsp extra-virgin olive oil
- 1 tbsp lemon juice
- 1 tbsp fresh parsley, chopped

Servings: Serves 4

Mode of cooking: No cooking required

Procedure:

In a large bowl, combine chickpeas, cherry tomatoes, cucumber, red onion, and Kalamata olives. Drizzle with olive oil and lemon juice, and toss gently to coat. Sprinkle with fresh parsley before serving.

Nutritional values: Approximately 260 calories | 11g protein | 10g fat | 34g carbohydrates

Recipe 2: Grilled Chicken and Quinoa Salad

Preparation time: 25 minutes

Ingredients:

- 2 boneless, skinless chicken breasts
- 1 cup cooked quinoa
- 2 cups mixed salad greens
- 1 cup cherry tomatoes, halved
- 1/2 cup cucumber, diced
- 1/4 cup feta cheese, crumbled
- 2 tbsp balsamic vinegar
- 1 tbsp extra-virgin olive oil

Servings: Serves 2

Mode of cooking: Grilling

Procedure:

Preheat the grill to medium-high heat. Season chicken breasts with salt and pepper. Grill chicken for about 6-8 minutes per side, or until cooked through. Remove from heat and let it rest for a few minutes before slicing. In a large bowl, combine cooked quinoa, salad greens, cherry tomatoes, cucumber, and feta cheese. Drizzle with balsamic vinegar and olive oil, and toss gently to combine. Top with sliced grilled chicken and serve.

Nutritional values: Approximately 400 calories | 34g protein | 12g fat | 39g carbohydrates

Recipe 3: Spinach and Strawberry Salad

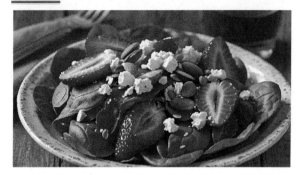

Preparation time: 10 minutes

Ingredients:

- 2 cups baby spinach
- 1 cup strawberries, sliced
- 1/4 cup sliced almonds
- 2 tbsp crumbled goat cheese
- 2 tbsp balsamic vinegar
- 1 tbsp extra-virgin olive oil

Servings: Serves 2

Mode of cooking: No cooking required

Procedure:

In a large bowl, combine baby spinach, sliced strawberries, sliced almonds, and crumbled goat cheese. Drizzle with balsamic vinegar and olive oil, and toss gently to coat.

Nutritional values: Approximately 180 calories | 8g protein | 13g fat | 9g carbohydrates

Recipe 4: Quinoa and Roasted Vegetable Salad

Preparation time: 30 minutes

Ingredients:

- 1 cup cooked quinoa
- 2 cups mixed roasted vegetables (such as bell peppers, zucchini, and eggplant), chopped
- 1/4 cup crumbled feta cheese
- 2 tbsp chopped fresh basil
- 2 tbsp lemon juice
- 1 tbsp extra-virgin olive oil

Servings: Serves 2

Mode of cooking: Roasting

Procedure:

Preheat the oven to 400°F (200°C). Toss mixed vegetables in olive oil, salt, and pepper, and spread them on a baking sheet. Roast vegetables for about 20 minutes, or until tender and slightly caramelized. In a large bowl, combine cooked quinoa, roasted vegetables, crumbled feta cheese, chopped fresh basil, lemon juice, and olive oil. Toss gently to combine.

Nutritional values: Approximately 290 calories | 11g protein | 8g fat | 44g carbohydrates

Recipe 5: Tuna and White Bean Salad

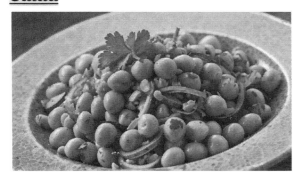

Preparation time: 15 minutes

Ingredients:

- 1 can (5 oz) tuna, drained
- 1 can (15 oz) white beans, rinsed and drained
- 1/2 red onion, diced
- 1/4 cup chopped fresh parsley
- 2 tbsp lemon juice
- 1 tbsp extra-virgin olive oil

Servings: Serves 4

Mode of cooking: No cooking required

Procedure:

In a large bowl, combine tuna, white beans, diced red onion, and chopped fresh parsley. Drizzle with lemon juice and olive oil, and toss gently to combine.

Nutritional values: Approximately 190 calories | 19g protein | 5g fat | 18g carbohydrates

---

4.2.2 Light Soups: Comforting Broths and Pureed Varieties

Recipe 1: Butternut Squash Soup

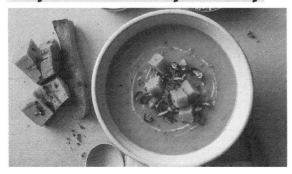

Preparation time: 40 minutes

Ingredients:

- 1 medium butternut squash, peeled, seeded, and diced
- 1 onion, diced
- 2 cloves garlic, minced
- 4 cups low-sodium vegetable broth
- 1/2 tsp ground ginger
- Salt and pepper to taste

Servings: Serves 6

Mode of cooking: Stovetop

Procedure:

In a large pot, sauté the onion and garlic until softened. Add the diced butternut squash, vegetable broth, ground ginger, salt, and pepper. Bring to a boil, then reduce heat and simmer for about 20-25 minutes until the squash is tender. Using an immersion blender, puree the soup until smooth.

Nutritional values: Approximately 120 calories | 2g protein | 1g fat | 28g carbohydrates

---

Recipe 2: Lentil Soup

Preparation time: 45 minutes

Ingredients:

- 1 cup dried brown lentils, rinsed
- 1 carrot, diced
- 1 celery stalk, diced
- 1 onion, diced
- 4 cups low-sodium chicken or vegetable broth
- 1 tsp cumin
- 1/2 tsp turmeric
- Salt and pepper to taste

Servings: Serves 4

Mode of cooking: Stovetop

Procedure:

In a large pot, combine the lentils, carrot, celery, onion, broth, cumin, turmeric, salt, and pepper. Bring to a boil, then reduce heat and simmer for about 30-35 minutes or until the lentils and vegetables are tender. Use an immersion blender to partially puree the soup, leaving some lentils and vegetables whole for texture.

Nutritional values: Approximately 220 calories | 15g protein | 1g fat | 40g carbohydrates

---

Recipe 3: Chicken and Vegetable Broth

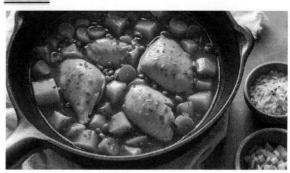

Preparation time: 1 hour

Ingredients:

- 2 bone-in, skinless chicken breasts
- 8 cups water
- 2 carrots, chopped
- 2 celery stalks, chopped
- 1 onion, chopped
- 2 garlic cloves, smashed
- 1 bay leaf
- Salt and pepper to taste

Servings: Serves 6

Mode of cooking: Stovetop

Procedure:

In a large pot, combine chicken breasts, water, carrots, celery, onion, garlic, bay leaf, salt, and pepper. Bring to a boil, then reduce heat and simmer for about 40-45 minutes or until the chicken is cooked through. Remove the chicken, shred the meat, and return it to the broth.

Nutritional values: Approximately 90 calories | 10g protein | 2g fat | 6g carbohydrates

Recipe 4: Potato Leek Soup

Preparation time: 50 minutes

Ingredients:

- 3 leeks, white and light green parts only, sliced
- 3 large potatoes, peeled and diced
- 4 cups low-sodium vegetable broth
- 1/2 cup unsweetened almond milk
- 1 tbsp olive oil

Servings: Serves 3

Mode of cooking: Stovetop

Procedure:

In a large pot, sauté the leeks in olive oil until softened. Add the diced potatoes and vegetable broth. Bring to a boil, then reduce heat and simmer for about 20-25 minutes until the potatoes are tender. Use an immersion blender to puree the soup until smooth, then stir in the almond milk.

Nutritional values: Approximately 180 calories | 5g protein | 4g fat | 30g carbohydrates

Recipe 5: Spinach and White Bean Soup

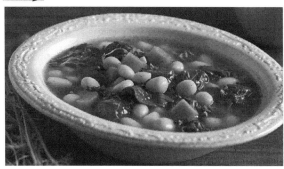

Preparation time: 35 minutes

Ingredients:

- 2 cups chopped spinach
- 1 can (15 oz) white beans, rinsed and drained
- 1 carrot, diced
- 1 celery stalk, diced
- 1 onion, diced
- 4 cups low-sodium vegetable broth
- 1 tsp dried thyme
- Salt and pepper to taste

Servings: Serves 4

Mode of cooking: Stovetop

Procedure:

In a large pot, combine the spinach, white beans, carrot, celery, onion, broth, thyme, salt, and pepper. Bring to a boil, then reduce heat and simmer for about 15-20 minutes until the vegetables are tender.

Nutritional values: Approximately 150 calories | 9g protein | 1g fat | 27g carbohydrates

4.2.3 Sandwiches and Wraps: Balanced, Digestion-Friendly Lunches

Recipe 1: Turkey and Avocado Wrap

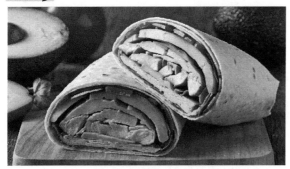

Preparation time = 15 minutes

Ingredients =

- 4 oz cooked turkey breast slices
- 1/2 avocado, sliced
- 1 whole wheat wrap

Servings = Serves 1

Mode of cooking: Assemble

Procedure:

Lay the whole wheat wrap flat on a clean surface. Place the turkey slices and avocado slices down the center of the wrap. Roll the wrap tightly, tucking in the sides as you go. Slice in half and serve.

Nutritional values: Approximately 350 calories | 25g protein | 10g fat | 35g carbohydrates

Recipe 2: Hummus and Veggie Sandwich

Preparation time = 10 minutes

Ingredients = 2 tbsp hummus

- 1/2 cucumber, thinly sliced
- 1/4 red bell pepper, sliced
- 2 slices whole grain bread

Servings = Serves 1

Mode of cooking: Assemble

Procedure:

Spread hummus on one slice of bread. Layer cucumber and red bell pepper slices on top of the hummus. Top with the second slice of bread. Cut in half and enjoy.

Nutritional values: Approximately 250 calories | 9g protein | 5g fat | 40g carbohydrates

Recipe 3: Tuna Salad Lettuce Wraps

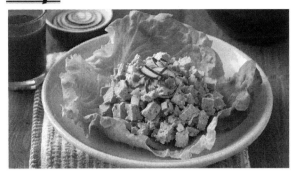

Preparation time = 20 minutes

Ingredients

- 1 can (5 oz) tuna, drained
- 1/4 cup diced celery
- 1/4 cup diced red onion
- 2 tbsp plain Greek yogurt
- Lettuce leaves (for wrapping)

Servings = Serves 2

Mode of cooking: Assemble

Procedure:

In a bowl, mix the tuna, celery, red onion, and Greek yogurt until well combined. Spoon the tuna salad on lettuce leaves and wrap to form lettuce wraps.

Nutritional values: Approximately 150 calories | 20g protein | 2g fat | 10g carbohydrates

Recipe 4: Egg Salad Sandwich

Preparation time = 20 minutes

Ingredients

- hard boiled eggs , chopped
- 2 tbsp plain Greek yogurt
- | ¼ cup diced cucumber
- | 2 slice whole grain bread

Procedure:

In a bowl, combine the chopped eggs, Greek yogurt, and diced cucumber. Spread the egg salad mixture on one slice of bread and top with the second slice.

Cut in half and serve.

Nutritional values: Approximately 280 calories | 20g protein | 10g fat | 25g carbohydrates

Recipe 5: Caprese Wrap

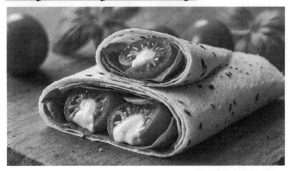

Preparation time = 10 minutes

Ingredients =

- 1 whole wheat wrap 1/2 cup cherry tomatoes,
- halved 2 oz
- fresh mozzarella, sliced Fresh basil leaves

Servings = Serves 1

Mode of cooking: Assemble

Procedure:

Lay the whole wheat wrap flat on a clean surface. Layer cherry tomatoes, fresh mozzarella slices, and basil leaves down the center of the wrap. Roll the wrap tightly and slice in half to serve.

Nutritional values: Approximately 300 calories | 15g protein | 15g fat | 30g carbohydrates

4.2.4 Bowls: Wholesome Lunch Bowls with Digestion-Supporting Ingredients

Recipe 1: Quinoa and Chicken Bowl

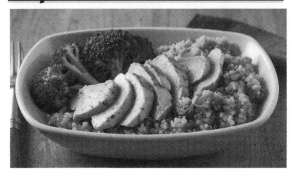

Preparation time = 30 minutes

Ingredients =

- 1 cup cooked quinoa
- 4 oz cooked chicken breast, sliced
- 1 cup steamed broccoli florets

Servings = Serves 2

Mode of cooking: Stovetop, steaming

Procedure:

Divide the cooked quinoa between two bowls. Top with the sliced chicken breast and steamed broccoli florets.

Nutritional values: Approximately 350 calories | 30g protein | 6g fat | 40g carbohydrates

Recipe 2: Sweet Potato and Black Bean Bowl

Preparation time = 40 minutes

Ingredients =

- 1 medium sweet potato,
- diced and roasted
- 1 cup cooked black beans
- 1/4 cup diced red bell pepper

Servings = Serves 2

Mode of cooking: Oven, stovetop

Procedure:

Divide the roasted sweet potato and cooked black beans between two bowls. Sprinkle with diced red bell pepper.

Nutritional values: Approximately 300 calories | 12g protein | 2g fat | 60g carbohydrates

Recipe 3: Salmon and Brown Rice Bowl

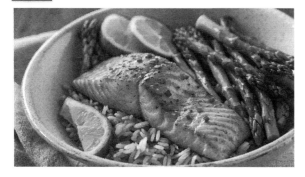

Preparation time = 25 minutes

- **Ingredients** = 8 oz grilled salmon filet
- 1 cup cooked brown rice
- 1 cup steamed asparagus

Servings = Serves 2

Mode of cooking: Grill, stovetop, steaming

Procedure:

Place the cooked brown rice in the bottom of two bowls. Top with grilled salmon and steamed asparagus.

Nutritional values: Approximately 400 calories | 35g protein | 15g fat | 30g carbohydrates

Recipe 4: Tofu and Vegetable Quinoa Bowl

Preparation time = 35 minutes

- **Ingredients** = 1 cup cooked quinoa
- 6 oz firm tofu, cubed and sautéed
- 1 cup mixed steamed vegetables (such as carrots, snap peas, and bell peppers)

Servings = Serves 2

Mode of cooking: Stovetop, steaming

Procedure:

Divide the cooked quinoa between two bowls.

Top with sautéed tofu and mixed steamed vegetables.

Nutritional values: Approximately 320 calories | 20g protein | 10g fat | 40g carbohydrates

Recipe 5: Shrimp and Zucchini Noodle Bowl

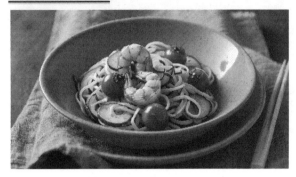

Preparation time = 20 minutes

Ingredients

- 8 oz cooked shrimp
- 2 medium zucchinis, spiralized and sautéed
- 1/4 cup cherry tomatoes, halved

Servings = Serves 2

Mode of cooking: Stovetop

Procedure:

Divide the sautéed zucchini noodles between two bowls. Top with cooked shrimp and cherry tomatoes.

Nutritional values: Approximately 250 calories | 25g protein | 5g fat | 20g carbohydrates

4.3 Dinners for Optimal Gut Health

When it comes to managing diverticulitis through diet, dinners play a crucial role in providing optimal gut health. In this chapter, we will explore a variety of recipes that are not only delicious but also gentle on the digestive system. These recipes are designed to promote healing and reduce the risk of triggering painful flare-ups, ensuring that you can enjoy your meals without compromising your health.

The Importance of Balanced Dinners

A well-balanced dinner is essential for individuals with diverticulitis. It should consist of a combination of lean proteins, healthy fats, and fiber-rich vegetables. Including these vital components in your meals can support the healing process and aid in digestion.

Lean Proteins for Gut Health

Proteins are the building blocks of our body, and they play a significant role in gut health. Opting for lean proteins such as grilled chicken, turkey, fish, and tofu can provide essential nutrients without putting excessive strain on the digestive system. These protein sources are easier to digest, making them ideal for individuals managing diverticulitis.

The Power of Healthy Fats

Contrary to popular belief, not all fats are bad for you. In fact, incorporating healthy fats into your diet can have numerous benefits for gut health. Avocado, olive oil, and nuts are excellent sources of monounsaturated fats, which can help reduce inflammation in the digestive tract. These fats contribute to a feeling of satiety and can be incorporated into your dinner recipes to enhance both flavor and nutrition.

Fiber: Essential for Digestion

Fiber is widely recognized as crucial for maintaining a healthy digestive system. However, it's important to choose the right types of fiber for individuals with diverticulitis. Insoluble fiber found in whole grains, fruits, and vegetables can be harsh on the colon and may increase the risk of flare-ups. Instead, focus on soluble fiber sources such as cooked vegetables, oatmeal, and certain fruits like bananas and applesauce. Soluble fiber is gentler on the digestive system and can aid in regular bowel movements without causing discomfort.

4.3.1 Grilled and Baked Proteins: Gentle and Satisfying Main Courses

Recipe 1: Herbed Baked Chicken Breast

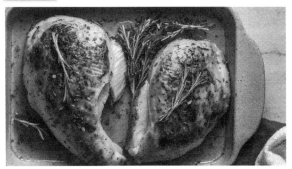

Preparation time: 30 minutes

Ingredients:

- 4 Chicken Breasts (about 6-8 ounces each)
- 2 tablespoons Olive Oil
- 3 cloves Garlic, minced
- 2 tablespoons Fresh Herbs (Rosemary & Thyme), finely chopped
- Salt and Pepper, to taste

Servings: 4

Mode of cooking: Baked

Procedure:

Preheat the oven to 375°F. Rub chicken breast with olive oil, minced garlic, and chopped fresh herbs. Bake for 25-30 minutes or until cooked through.

Nutritional values: 250 calories | 30g protein | 12g fat | 2g carbohydrates

Recipe 2: Lemon Herb Baked Salmon

Preparation time: 25 minutes

Ingredients:

- 2 Salmon Fillets (6-ounces each)
- 2 tablespoons Olive Oil
- 1 Lemon (half for juice, half sliced for garnish)
- 2 tablespoons Fresh Dill, finely chopped
- Salt and Pepper, to taste

Servings: 2

Mode of cooking: Baked

Procedure:

Preheat the oven to 400°F. Place salmon filets on a baking sheet, drizzle with olive oil, squeeze lemon juice, and add chopped dill. Bake for 15-20 minutes.

Nutritional values: 300 calories | 25g protein | 18g fat | 3g carbohydrates

Recipe 3: Rosemary Garlic Grilled Shrimp

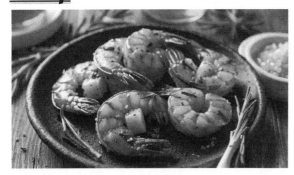

Preparation time: 20 minutes

Ingredients:

- 1 pound Large Shrimp, peeled and deveined (approx. 20-24 shrimp)
- 3 cloves Garlic, minced
- 2 tablespoons Fresh Rosemary, finely chopped
- 3 tablespoons Olive Oil
- Salt and Pepper, to taste

Servings: 3

Mode of cooking: Grilled

Procedure:

Marinate shrimp in minced garlic, chopped rosemary, and olive oil. Grill on skewers until pink and cooked.

Nutritional values: 180 calories | 20g protein | 8g fat | 5g carbohydrates

Recipe 4: Baked Lemon Herb Tofu

Preparation time: 35 minutes

Ingredients:

- 1 block (14-16 ounces) Extra Firm Tofu
- 2 Lemons (1 for juice, 1 sliced for garnish)
- 1/4 cup Fresh Parsley, finely chopped
- 3 tablespoons Olive Oil
- Salt and Pepper, to taste

Servings: 4

Mode of cooking: Baked

Procedure:

Press tofu, then marinate in lemon juice, chopped parsley, and olive oil. Bake at 375°F for 25-30 minutes.

Nutritional values: 200 calories | 15g protein | 12g fat | 10g carbohydrates

Recipe 5: Ginger Soy Baked Turkey Meatballs

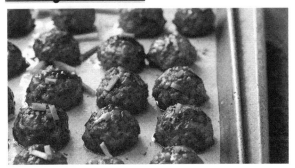

Preparation time: 40 minutes

Ingredients:

- 1.5 pounds Ground Turkey
- 2 tablespoons Ginger, fresh and minced
- 1/4 cup Soy Sauce
- 1/2 cup Green Onions, finely chopped
- Salt and Pepper, to taste

Servings: 6

Mode of cooking: Baked

Procedure:

Mix ground turkey with minced ginger, soy sauce, and chopped green onions. Form into meatballs and bake at 400°F for 20-25 minutes.

Nutritional values: 180 calories | 24g protein | 8g fat | 4g carbohydrates

4.3.2 Vegetable Sides: Steamed and Roasted Options for Gut Health

Recipe 1: Lemon Roasted Broccoli

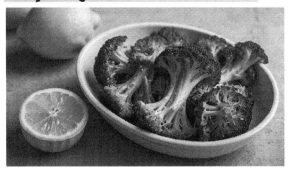

Preparation time: 25 minutes

Ingredients:

- 1.5 pounds Broccoli Florets
- 2 tablespoons Olive Oil
- 3 cloves Garlic, minced
- Zest of 1 Lemon
- Juice of 1 Lemon
- Salt, to taste

Servings: 4

Mode of cooking: Roasted

Procedure:

Preheat the oven to 425°F. Toss broccoli florets with olive oil, minced garlic, and lemon zest. Roast for 15-20 minutes or until tender and crispy. Sprinkle it with lemon juice and salt.

Nutritional values: 70 calories | 3g protein | 4g fat | 8g carbohydrates

Recipe 2: Steamed Carrots and Green Beans

Preparation time: 20 minutes

Ingredients:

- 1 pound Carrots, peeled and cut into bite-sized pieces
- 1 pound Green Beans, trimmed and cut into bite-sized pieces
- 2 tablespoons Butter
- Salt, to taste

Servings: 4

Mode of cooking: Steamed

Procedure:

Trim and cut carrots and green beans into bite-sized pieces. Steam for 10-12 minutes or until tender. Toss with butter and salt.

Nutritional values: 50 calories | 2g protein | 3g fat | 9g carbohydrates

Recipe 3: Roasted Brussels Sprouts with Parmesan

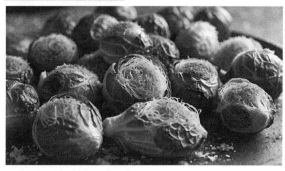

Preparation time: 30 minutes

Ingredients:

- 1 pound Brussels Sprouts, trimmed and halved
- 2 tablespoons Olive Oil
- 1/4 cup Parmesan Cheese, grated
- Salt, to taste

Servings: 4

Mode of cooking: Roasted

Procedure: Preheat oven to 400°F. Toss trimmed Brussels sprouts with olive oil and salt, roast for 20-25 minutes or until crispy. Sprinkle with grated Parmesan cheese.

Nutritional values: 90 calories | 7g protein | 5g fat | 8g carbohydrates

Recipe 4: Garlic Roasted Zucchini and Squash

Preparation time: 25 minutes

Ingredients:

- 2 medium Zucchinis
- 2 medium Yellow Squashes
- 3 cloves Garlic, minced
- 3 tablespoons Olive Oil
- Salt, to taste

Servings: 4

Mode of cooking: Roasted

Procedure:

Preheat the oven to 400°F. Cut zucchini and squash into half-inch rounds, toss with minced garlic and olive oil, and sprinkle with salt. Roast for 15-20 minutes, until tender.

Nutritional values: 60 calories | 2g protein | 4g fat | 6g carbohydrates

Recipe 5: Steamed Asparagus with Lemon Butter

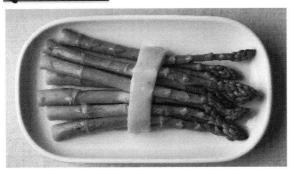

Preparation time: 20 minutes

Ingredients:

- 1 pound Asparagus
- 2 tablespoons Butter
- 1 tablespoon Lemon Juice
- Salt, to taste

Servings: 4

Mode of cooking: Steamed

Procedure:

Snap off the tough ends of the asparagus. Steam for 5-7 minutes or until tender. Toss with melted butter, lemon juice, and salt.

Nutritional values: 40 calories | 2g protein | 4g fat | 2g carbohydrates

4.3.3 Casseroles: One-Dish Meals Made with Ease

Recipe 1: Turkey and Quinoa Casserole

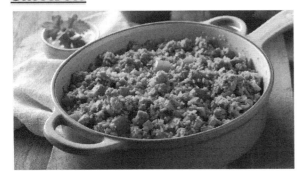

Preparation time: 45 minutes

Ingredients:

- 1 cup Quinoa, uncooked
- 1 pound Ground Turkey
- 1 medium Onion, chopped
- 1 Bell Pepper, diced (any color)
- Salt, to taste
- Pepper, to taste
- Optional: shredded cheese, herbs, or spices for additional flavor

Servings: 6

Mode of cooking: Baked

Procedure:

Cook quinoa according to package instructions. In a skillet, cook ground turkey with diced bell peppers and onions. Combine cooked quinoa and turkey mixture in a baking dish. Bake at 375°F for 25-30 minutes.

Nutritional values: 300 calories | 25g protein | 10g fat | 25g carbohydrates

Recipe 2: Sweet Potato and Lentil Casserole

Preparation time: 50 minutes

Ingredients:

- 2 large Sweet Potatoes, peeled and thinly sliced
- 1 cup Lentils, rinsed
- 4 cups Spinach, fresh
- 3 cloves Garlic, minced
- Salt and Pepper, to taste
- Olive oil, for drizzling (optional)

Servings: 4

Mode of cooking: Baked

Procedure:

Boil lentils until tender. Layer sliced sweet potatoes, cooked lentils, and spinach in a baking dish. Sprinkle with minced garlic and bake at 400°F for 35-40 minutes.

Nutritional values: 250 calories | 15g protein | 5g fat | 40g carbohydrates

Recipe 3: Chicken and Brown Rice Casserole

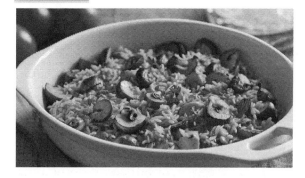

Preparation time: 55 minutes

Ingredients:

- 2 Chicken Breasts, diced
- 1 cup Brown Rice, uncooked
- 2 cups Chicken Broth
- 2 cups Mushrooms, sliced
- Salt and Pepper, to taste
- Olive oil or Cooking Spray

Servings: 5

Mode of cooking: Baked

Procedure:

Cook brown rice in chicken broth. Sauté sliced mushrooms and diced chicken breast. Combine cooked rice, chicken, and mushrooms in a casserole dish. Bake at 350°F for 30-35 minutes.

Nutritional values: 280 calories | 20g protein | 7g fat | 35g carbohydrates

Recipe 4: Spinach and Ricotta Zucchini Casserole

Preparation time: 40 minutes

Ingredients:

- 4 Zucchinis, medium-sized, thinly sliced
- 2 cups Spinach, fresh (can use frozen, thawed and drained if fresh is not available)
- 1 cup Ricotta Cheese
- 2 Eggs, beaten
- Salt and Pepper, to taste
- Non-stick Cooking Spray or Olive Oil

Servings: 4

Mode of cooking: Baked

Procedure:

Slice zucchini and layer with cooked spinach in a baking dish. Mix ricotta cheese with beaten eggs and pour over the zucchini and spinach. Bake at 375°F for 25-30 minutes.

Nutritional values: 220 calories | 15g protein | 10g fat | 18g carbohydrates

Recipe 5: Butternut Squash and Black Bean Casserole

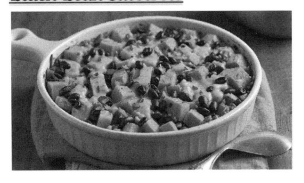

Preparation time: 50 minutes

Ingredients:

- 1 medium Butternut Squash (about 2 pounds), peeled, seeded, and cut into 1-inch cubes
- 2 cups Black Beans, cooked or canned (if canned, drain and rinse)
- 1 tsp Cumin
- 1 large Onion, diced
- Salt and Pepper, to taste
- Cooking Oil Spray or Olive Oil
- Cilantro or Parsley (optional), chopped for garnish

Servings: 6

Mode of cooking: Baked

Procedure:

Roast butternut squash until tender. Sauté diced onions and cumin, then mix with black beans. Layer squash and bean mixture in a baking dish. Bake at 375°F for 30-35 minutes.

Nutritional values: 230 calories | 12g protein | 3g fat | 40g carbohydrates

4.3.4 Stir-Fries: Quick and Customizable for a Gentle Evening Meal

Recipe 1: Shrimp and Vegetable Stir-Fry

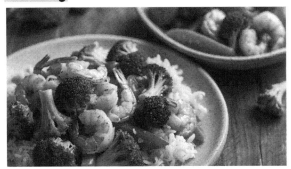

Preparation time: 20 minutes

Ingredients:

- 8 oz Shrimp, peeled and deveined
- 1 Bell Pepper, sliced into strips
- 2 cups Broccoli Florets
- 2 cloves Garlic, minced
- 1 Tbsp Cooking Oil (such as vegetable oil or canola oil)
- Salt and Pepper, to taste
- Soy sauce or Stir-Fry Sauce

- (optional, for flavor)
- Cooked rice or noodles for serving (optional)

Servings: 2

Mode of cooking: Stir-fried

Procedure:

Sauté shrimp, bell peppers, and broccoli in a hot skillet with minced garlic until shrimp is cooked and vegetables are crisp-tender. Serve hot.

Nutritional values: 200 calories | 25g protein | 5g fat | 15g carbohydrates

Recipe 2: Chicken and Snow Pea Stir-Fry

Preparation time: 25 minutes

Ingredients:

- 8 oz Chicken Breast, thinly sliced
- 1 cup Snow Peas
- 1 large Carrot, julienned
- 2 Tbsp Soy Sauce
- 1 Tbsp Cooking Oil (such as vegetable or canola oil)
- Salt and Pepper, to taste
- Cooked rice or noodles for serving (optional)

Servings: 2

Mode of cooking: Stir-fried

Procedure:

Stir-fry thinly sliced chicken breast until cooked. Add snow peas and julienned carrots, and continue stir-frying until vegetables are tender-crisp. Season with soy sauce and serve hot.

Nutritional values: 250 calories | 30g protein | 6g fat | 20g carbohydrates

Recipe 3: Tofu and Bok Choy Stir-Fry

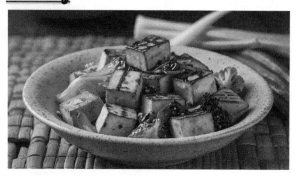

Preparation time: 30 minutes

Ingredients:

- 14 oz Tofu (firm or extra firm), drained and cubed
- 2 cups Bok Choy, chopped
- 1 cup Mushrooms, sliced (any variety)
- 1 Tbsp Ginger, grated
- 2 Tbsp Cooking Oil (such as vegetable or sesame oil)
- Soy Sauce to taste (optional)
- Salt and Pepper, to taste
- Cooked rice or noodles for serving (optional)

Servings: 2

Mode of cooking: Stir-fried

Procedure:

Stir-fry cubed tofu, chopped bok choy, sliced mushrooms, and grated ginger until tofu is golden and vegetables are tender. Serve hot.

Nutritional values: 180 calories | 20g

protein | 8g fat | 10g carbohydrates

Recipe 4: Beef and Asparagus Stir-Fry

Preparation time: 25 minutes

Ingredients:

- 8 oz Beef Sirloin, thinly sliced
- 2 cups Asparagus, trimmed and cut into 1-inch pieces
- 1 medium Red Onion, thinly sliced
- 2 Tbsp Sesame Oil
- Soy Sauce to taste (optional)
- Salt and Pepper, to taste
- Cooked rice or noodles for serving (optional)

Servings: 2

Mode of cooking: Stir-fried

Procedure:

Sauté thinly sliced beef sirloin, asparagus spears, and sliced red onion in sesame oil until beef is cooked and vegetables are crisp-tender. Serve hot.

Nutritional values: 300 calories | 25g protein | 15g fat | 15g carbohydrates

Recipe 5: Mushroom and Spinach Stir-Fry

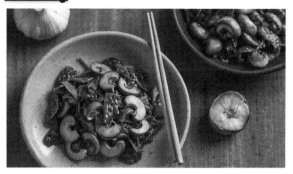

Preparation time: 20 minutes

Ingredients:

- 2 cups Mushrooms, sliced (any variety)
- 3 cups Spinach, fresh
- 2 cloves Garlic, minced
- 2 Tbsp Olive Oil
- Salt and Pepper, to taste
- Cooked quinoa, rice, or whole grains for serving (optional)

Servings: 2

Mode of cooking: Stir-fried

Procedure: Sauté sliced mushrooms and minced garlic in olive oil until mushrooms are tender. Add spinach and stir until wilted. Serve hot.

Nutritional values: 150 calories | 8g protein | 7g fat | 15g carbohydrates

4.4 Snacks and Mini-Meals: Eating Well Between Meals

A diagnosis of diverticulitis can be disconcerting, prompting a step back and an evaluation of dietary habits. Apart from major meals, it's critical to focus on how we fuel our bodies when hunger pangs strike during the day's odd hours. Casually snacking might seem insignificant, but the food choices we make during these times have a substantial impact. Let's dive into the art of crafting snacks and mini-meals, which are flavorful, nutritive, and gentle on a delicate digestive system.

The Essential Role of Snacks and Mini-Meals

Snacking serves multiple purposes in a diverticulitis-friendly diet plan. By providing nutrient-dense food options, we ensure sustained energy levels and curb the temptation to overindulge during main meals, lightening the load on our digestive systems.

However, these must not merely be mindless fillers. To truly make a positive impact, carefully chosen or crafted snacks can function as small but potent powerhouses of nutrition to complement your primary meals.

Hummus - the Wholesome Dip

Homemade hummus, the creamy Middle Eastern dip, emerges as a superb candidate for our cause. Packed with protein and fiber and virtually fat-free, its primary ingredient, chickpeas, deliver vital nutrients without overwhelming the gut.

To add variety, team your hummus with different crudités such as tender cucumber or bell pepper strips for a refreshing change. The crisp crunch, vibrant colors and benefit of additional nutrients transform a mundane snack into one you eagerly look forward to.

Invincible Smoothies: Tailor-made Nutrition in a Glass

Smoothies offer unparalleled versatility, allowing us myriad combinations and control over the nutritional content. Select fruits and vegetables, pureed to smooth consistency, make smoothies a dream option for a gut taking baby steps towards healing. A leisurely morning or a mid-afternoon energy slump, you can whip up a fruit smoothie tailored to your taste and needs.

Imagine welcoming a day with a deep golden smoothie made of fully ripe banana puree, cooked apple compote, and a dollop of creamy yogurt. This concoction is a treasure trove of soluble fiber, excellent for bowel health, plus the probiotics from the yogurt promoting robust gut flora.

Broths to Boost Wellness

Nourishment and comfort flow in equal measures from a steaming bowl of soup or broth. The charm of soup lies in the breakdown of food pieces to tiny fractions. This small size facilitates maximum nutrient absorption and exerts the least strain on your digestive system. All the hydration benefits, the essential minerals, and the warmth of soup come without imposing a digestive burden.

Optimizing Popcorn for Diverticulitis

Whole grains aren't typically recommended for diverticulitis, popcorn is a worthy exception if appropriately managed. Fully popped popcorn, without any hard kernels or hulls, is a good snack option.

In the next section you will find some enjoyable snack recipes.

4.4.1 Healthy Fats and Nuts: Small Portions for Sustained Energy

Recipe 1: Roasted Carrots with Ginger

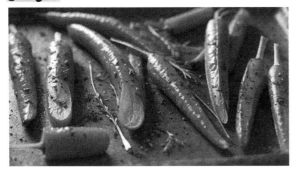

Preparation time = 10 minutes

Ingredients

- 4-5 carrots, peeled and sliced
- 1 tablespoon olive oil
- 1 teaspoon grated fresh ginger |
- Salt and pepper to taste

Servings = Serves 2

Mode of cooking: Oven

Procedure:

Preheat the oven to 400 degrees Fahrenheit. Toss carrots with olive oil, ginger, salt, and pepper in a bowl. Spread carrots on a baking sheet and roast for 20-25 minutes or until tender when pierced with a fork.

Nutritional values: 97 calories | 2g protein | 4g fat | 17g carbohydrates

---

Recipe 2: Tuna and Vegetable Salad

Preparation time = 15 minutes

Ingredients

- 1 can of tuna in water, drained
- 1/2 cucumber, diced
- 1/2 red bell pepper, diced
- 1/2 onion, diced
- 1 tablespoon olive oil
- Salt and pepper to taste

Servings = Serves 2

Mode of cooking: No Cooking Required

Procedure:

In a bowl, mix together tuna, cucumber,

red bell pepper, and onion. Drizzle with olive oil and season with salt and pepper to taste.

Nutritional values: 225 calories | 20g protein | 8g fat | 18g carbohydrates

Recipe 3: Greek Yogurt and Fruit Parfait

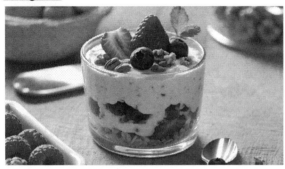

Preparation time = 10 minutes

Ingredients

- 1/2 cup Greek yogurt
- 1/4 cup chopped mixed fruit (such as strawberries, blueberries, and raspberries)
- 1 tablespoon honey
- 2 tablespoons chopped walnuts

Servings = Serves 1

Mode of cooking: No Cooking Required

Procedure:

In a glass, layer Greek yogurt, mixed fruit, and honey. Top with chopped walnuts before serving.

Nutritional values: 249 calories | 17g protein | 11g fat | 24g carbohydrates

Recipe 4: Grilled Chicken and Vegetable Skewers

Preparation time = 30 minutes (including marinating time)

Ingredients

- 1 boneless, skinless chicken breast, cut into cubes
- 1/2 zucchini, sliced
- 1/2 red onion, sliced
- 1/2 red bell pepper, sliced
- 1 tablespoon olive oil
- 1 tablespoon fresh lemon juice |
- 1 teaspoon dried oregano
- Salt and pepper to taste

Servings = Serves 2

Mode of cooking: Grill or stovetop

Procedure:

In a bowl, mix together olive oil, lemon juice, oregano, salt, and pepper. Add chicken cubes and vegetables, toss and marinate for 10-15 minutes. Skewer chicken and vegetables on wooden or metal skewers and grill or cook on stovetop until chicken is cooked through.

Nutritional values: 214 calories | 27g protein | 9g fat | 8g carbohydrates

Recipe 5: Sweet Potato and Black Bean Salad

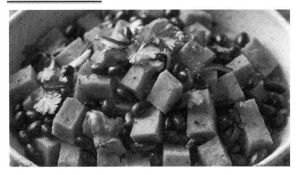

Preparation time = 20 minutes

Ingredients

- 2 medium sweet potatoes, peeled and diced
- 1 can black beans, rinsed and drained
- 1/2 red onion, diced
- 1/2 red bell pepper, diced
- 1 tablespoon olive oil
- 1 tablespoon fresh lime juice
- 1/2 teaspoon ground cumin
- Salt and pepper to taste

Servings = Serves 2

Mode of cooking: Oven

Procedure:

Preheat the oven to 400 degrees Fahrenheit. Toss sweet potatoes with olive oil, cumin, salt, and pepper in a bowl. Spread sweet potatoes on a baking sheet and roast for 20-25 minutes or until tender when pierced with a fork. In a serving bowl, mix together sweet potatoes, black beans, red onion, red bell pepper, lime juice, and additional salt and pepper to taste.

Nutritional values: 318 calories | 10g protein | 6g fat | 56g carbohydrates

4.4.2 Fruit-Based Snacks: Gentle on the Digestive System

Recipe 1: Berry Chia Pudding

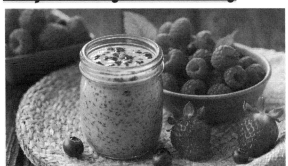

Preparation time = 5 minutes (plus chilling time)

Ingredients

- 1 cup mixed berries (such as strawberries, blueberries, and raspberries)
- 1 cup unsweetened almond milk
- 2 tablespoons chia seeds
- 1 tablespoon honey or maple syrup (optional)

Servings = Serves 1

Mode of cooking: No Cooking Required

Procedure:

In a jar or bowl, mash the mixed berries with a fork. Add almond milk, chia seeds, and optional honey or maple syrup. Stir well to combine. Cover and refrigerate for at least 2 hours or overnight until the mixture thickens, resembling a pudding-like consistency.

Nutritional values: 197 calories | 5g protein | 9g fat | 25g carbohydrates

Recipe 2: Apple Slices with Almond Butter

Preparation time = 5 minutes

Ingredients

- 1 apple, sliced
- 2 tablespoons almond butter

Servings = Serves 1

Mode of cooking: No Cooking Required

Procedure:

Slice the apple into thin slices. Spread almond butter on the apple slices.

Serve immediately.

Nutritional values: 237 calories | 5g protein | 14g fat | 26g carbohydrates

Recipe 3: Banana and Peanut Butter Smoothie

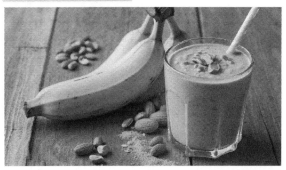

Preparation time = 5 minutes

Ingredients

- 1 ripe banana
- 1 cup unsweetened almond milk
- 2 tablespoons natural peanut butter
- 1 tablespoon honey (optional)

Servings = Serves 1

Mode of cooking: Blender

Procedure:

Peel the banana and place it in a blender. Add almond milk, peanut butter, and optional honey. Blend until smooth and creamy. Pour into a glass and serve chilled.

Nutritional values: 378 calories | 12g protein | 18g fat | 45g carbohydrates

Recipe 4: Citrus Fruit Salad

Preparation time = 10 minutes

Ingredients

- 1 orange, peeled and segmented
- 1 grapefruit, peeled and segmented
- 1 kiwi, peeled and sliced
- 1 tablespoon fresh lime juice
- 1 tablespoon honey

Servings = Serves 2

Mode of cooking: No Cooking Required

Procedure:

In a bowl, combine orange segments, grapefruit segments, and kiwi slices.

Drizzle with fresh lime juice and honey. Toss gently to coat all the fruit. Serve immediately or refrigerate until ready to serve.

Nutritional values: 174 calories | 2g protein | 0g fat | 43g carbohydrates

Recipe 5: Mango Coconut Yogurt Parfait

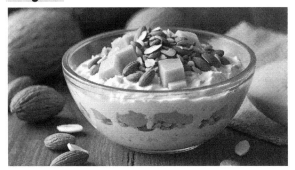

Preparation time = 10 minutes

Ingredients

- 1 ripe mango, peeled and diced
- 1 cup unsweetened coconut yogurt |
- 2 tablespoons shredded coconut
- 1 tablespoon chopped almonds

Servings = Serves 1

Mode of cooking: No Cooking Required

Procedure:

In a glass or jar, layer diced mango, coconut yogurt, shredded coconut, and chopped almonds. Repeat the layers until all ingredients are used. Top with additional mango and shredded coconut for garnish, if desired.

Nutritional values: 340 calories | 6g protein | 12g fat | 57g carbohydrates

4.4.3 Homemade Bars and Energy Balls: Nutrient-Packed Bites

Recipe 1: Almond Date Energy Bars

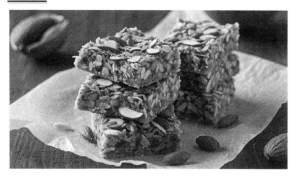

Preparation time = 15 minutes

Ingredients

- 1 cup pitted dates
- 1 cup almonds
- 1/4 cup unsweetened shredded coconut

Servings = Makes 8 bars

Mode of cooking: No Cooking Required

Procedure:

In a food processor, pulse dates, almonds, and shredded coconut until the mixture starts to come together. Transfer the mixture to a square or rectangular dish lined with parchment paper. Press the mixture firmly and evenly into the dish. Place in the refrigerator for at least 1 hour to set, then slice into bars.

Nutritional values: 199 calories | 5g protein | 11g fat | 24g carbohydrates

---

Recipe 2: No-Bake Oatmeal Energy Bites

Preparation time = 10 minutes (plus chilling time)

Ingredients

- 1 cup old-fashioned oats
- 1/2 cup natural peanut butter
- 1/4 cup honey
- 1/4 cup chopped nuts (such as walnuts or almonds)
- 1/4 cup mini chocolate chips

Servings = Makes 12 bites

Mode of cooking: No Cooking Required

Procedure:

In a bowl, mix together oats, peanut butter, honey, chopped nuts, and mini chocolate chips until well combined. Roll the mixture into tablespoon-sized balls and place them on a baking sheet. Chill in the refrigerator for at least 30 minutes before serving.

Nutritional values: 138 calories | 4g protein | 7g fat | 16g carbohydrates

---

Recipe 3: Cranberry Almond Protein Bars

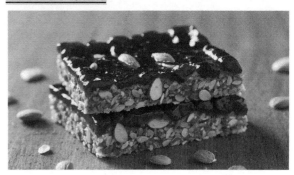

Preparation time = 20 minutes

Ingredients

- 1/2 cup almond butter
- 1/4 cup honey
- 1 1/2 cups rolled oats
- 1/2 cup chopped dried cranberries
- 1/4 cup chopped almonds

Servings = Makes 8 bars

Mode of cooking: No Cooking Required

Procedure:

In a microwave-safe bowl, combine almond butter and honey. Microwave for 30 seconds and stir until smooth. Stir in rolled oats, dried cranberries, and chopped almonds until well combined. Press the mixture into a square or rectangular dish lined with parchment paper and refrigerate for at least 1 hour before cutting into bars.

Nutritional values: 234 calories | 7g protein | 11g fat | 29g carbohydrates

Recipe 4: Apricot Coconut Energy Balls

Preparation time = 15 minutes

Ingredients

- 1 cup dried apricots
- 1 cup raw almonds
- 1/4 cup unsweetened shredded coconut

Servings = Makes 12 balls

Mode of cooking: No Cooking Required

Procedure:

In a food processor, blend dried apricots and raw almonds until the mixture starts to stick together. Roll the mixture into tablespoon-sized balls. Roll the balls in shredded coconut until coated. Refrigerate for 30 minutes before serving.

Nutritional values: 99 calories | 3g protein | 5g fat | 12g carbohydrates

Recipe 5: Pumpkin Seed Cocoa Bars

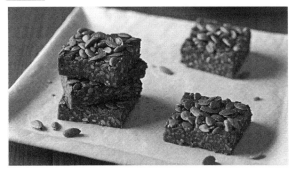

Preparation time = 25 minutes

Ingredients =

- 1/2 cup pumpkin seeds
- 1/4 cup cocoa powder
- 1/4 cup honey
- 1/4 cup almond butter
- 1/2 teaspoon vanilla extract

Servings = Makes 8 bars

Mode of cooking: No Cooking Required

Procedure:

In a food processor, pulse pumpkin seeds until finely chopped. Add cocoa powder, honey, almond butter, and vanilla extract. Process until the mixture forms a dough. Press the dough into a square or rectangular dish lined with parchment paper and refrigerate for at least 2 hours before cutting into bars.

Nutritional values

- 177 calories
- 5g protein
- 11g fat
- 17g carbohydrates

4.4.4 Yogurts and Probiotic-Rich Foods: Supporting Gut Flora

Recipe 1: Blueberry Yogurt Parfait

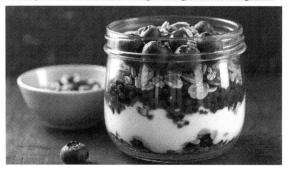

Preparation time = 5 minutes

Ingredients

- 1 cup plain Greek yogurt
- 1/2 cup fresh blueberries
- 1/4 cup granola
- 1 tablespoon honey

Servings = 1 serving

Mode of cooking: No Cooking Required

Procedure:

In a bowl or cup, layer yogurt, blueberries, and granola. Drizzle honey over the top.

Nutritional values: 347 calories | 23g protein | 9g fat | 45g carbohydrates

Recipe 2: Kimchi Fried Rice

Preparation time = 15 minutes

Ingredients =

- 1 cup cooked brown rice
- 1/2 cup chopped kimchi
- 1/4 cup chopped scallions
- 1 tablespoon sesame oil
- 1 teaspoon soy sauce

Servings = 1 serving

Mode of cooking: Stovetop

Procedure:

In a pan, heat sesame oil over medium heat. Add chopped kimchi and scallions, sautéing until fragrant. Add cooked brown rice and soy sauce, stir until well combined and heated through.

Nutritional values

- 424 calories
- 10g protein
- 15g fat
- 68g carbohydrates

Recipe 3: Avocado Toast with Sauerkraut

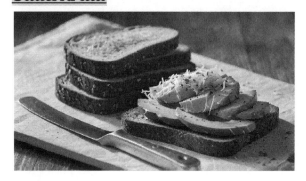

Preparation time = 5 minutes

Ingredients

- 1 slice of whole grain bread
- 1/2 avocado, sliced
- 1/4 cup sauerkraut

Servings = 1 serving

Mode of cooking: Toasting

Procedure:

Toast the slice of bread. Top the toasted bread with sliced avocado and sauerkraut.

Nutritional values: 329 calories | 7g protein | 18g fat | 33g carbohydrates

Recipe 4: Baked Sweet Potato with Yogurt and Chives

Preparation time = 1 hour

Ingredients

- 1 medium sweet potato
- 1/4 cup plain Greek yogurt
- 1 tablespoon chopped chives

Servings = 1 serving

Mode of cooking: Baking

Procedure:

Preheat the oven to 400°F. Pierce the sweet potato a few times with a fork and place it on a baking sheet. Bake for 45-60 minutes until the sweet potato is tender. Slice the sweet potato open and top with Greek yogurt and chopped chives.

Nutritional values: 284 calories | 13g protein | 1g fat | 63g carbohydrates

Recipe 5: Beet and Fennel Salad with Kefir Dressing

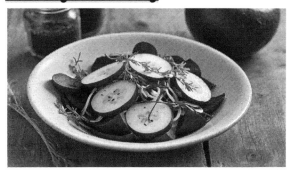

Preparation time = 15 minutes

Ingredients

- 1 medium beet
- 1/2 bulb fennel, sliced
- 1/4 cup plain kefir
- 1 tablespoon olive oil
- 1/2 tablespoon honey
- 1/2 tablespoon apple cider vinegar

Servings = 1 serving

Mode of cooking: No Cooking Required

Procedure:

Thinly slice the beet and fennel. In a bowl, whisk together kefir, olive oil, honey, and apple cider vinegar to make the dressing. Toss the salad with the dressing.

Nutritional values: 227 calories | 6g protein | 9g fat | 33g carbohydrates

4.5 Special Section: International Cuisine Diverticulitis-Friendly Dishes

Diet plays a crucial role in managing diverticulitis, and embracing international cuisine can add variety and flavor to your meals while adhering to diverticulitis-friendly guidelines. Global cuisines offer a rich tapestry of ingredients and flavors that can be adapted to suit a diverticulitis-friendly diet. Exploring international dishes can provide a diverse range of nutrients while minimizing the risk of triggering painful flare-ups.

Mediterranean Delights

The Mediterranean diet has long been celebrated for its health benefits, particularly its emphasis on fresh fruits, vegetables, whole grains, and healthy fats. For those with diverticulitis, the Mediterranean diet offers a colorful array of dishes that are gentle on the digestive system and abundant in essential nutrients. From Greek salads with tender lettuce, cucumbers, and olive oil to Italian vegetable risottos and Spanish seafood paella, Mediterranean cuisine offers a myriad of options that align with diverticulitis management. Embracing this cuisine can be a delightful journey into dishes that are not only flavorful but also supportive of gastrointestinal health.

Asian Inspirations

Incorporating Asian cuisine into your diverticulitis-friendly diet can introduce a wealth of aromatic herbs, spices, and wholesome ingredients. Japanese miso soups, Vietnamese pho with rice noodles, and stir-fried tofu with ginger and vegetables are just a few examples of Asian dishes that can add depth and variety to your menu without compromising your digestive health. Asian cuisines often feature an abundance of plant-based ingredients, lean proteins, and fermented foods, which can contribute to a well-rounded and gut-friendly diet.

Latin American Flavors

Latin American cuisine is a vibrant tapestry of flavors and textures that can be adapted to accommodate diverticulitis management. Dishes such as Brazilian black bean stew, Mexican chicken and vegetable fajitas, and Peruvian quinoa salad provide a fusion of colors and flavors that are not only delicious but also supportive of gastrointestinal well-being. Embracing Latin American cuisine can bring a sense of culinary adventure to your diverticulitis-friendly repertoire, offering a diverse selection of dishes to suit different tastes and preferences.

Middle Eastern Treasures

The Middle Eastern diet offers a treasure trove of dishes rich in fiber, beneficial fats, and wholesome ingredients that can support diverticulitis management. From creamy hummus and tabbouleh to grilled kebabs and lentil soups, Middle Eastern cuisine provides an array of options that cater to individuals seeking to maintain a balanced and gut-friendly diet. The use of ingredients such as chickpeas, lentils, whole grains, and a variety of herbs and spices adds depth and complexity to Middle Eastern dishes, enriching your culinary experience while promoting digestive wellness.

European Comforts

European cuisine, with its emphasis on hearty stews, roasted vegetables, and simple yet satisfying ingredients, can be adapted to align with diverticulitis-friendly guidelines. Dishes such as Irish colcannon, Spanish vegetable paella, and Italian minestrone soup offer a comforting embrace of flavors and textures while respecting the dietary needs of individuals managing diverticulitis. Exploring European cuisine can provide a sense of familiarity and comfort, ensuring that you can enjoy a variety of satisfying and nourishing dishes while safeguarding your digestive health.

When exploring international cuisines, it's important to be mindful of individual tolerances and dietary restrictions. Experimenting with different culinary traditions can add a touch of excitement and exploration to your diverticulitis-friendly journey, while broadening your palate and nutritional intake. Remember to incorporate these international dishes into your diet in moderation and ensure that they align with your specific dietary needs and the guidance of your healthcare provider. By embracing diverse global cuisines, you can expand your culinary horizons while nourishing your body with the wholesome, gut-friendly ingredients that support your journey toward digestive wellness.

4.5.1 Asian-Inspired Recipes: Flavorful Dishes with a Digestive Twist

In the quest for flavorful Asian-inspired dishes that align with diverticulitis-friendly dietary guidelines, the following collection of recipes provides a delightful array of options that are gentle on the digestive system while delivering vibrant, aromatic flavors. Each recipe has been carefully crafted to ensure that it combines nourishing ingredients that support digestive wellness.

Recipe 1: Miso-Ginger Glazed Salmon

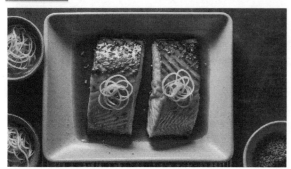

Preparation time = 20 minutes

Ingredients

- 4 Salmon Fillets
- 3 tablespoons Miso Paste
- 1 tablespoon Freshly Grated Ginger

Servings = Serves 4

Mode of cooking: Baking

Procedure:

Preheat the oven to 375°F (190°C). In a small bowl, mix 3 tablespoons of miso paste with 1 tablespoon of freshly grated ginger. Place the salmon filets on a baking sheet lined with parchment paper and spread the miso-ginger mixture over the top of each filet. Bake for 12-15 minutes, or until the salmon is cooked through and the glaze is golden brown.

Nutritional values: 329 calories | 34g protein | 18g fat | 1g carbohydrates

Recipe 2: Vietnamese-Inspired Shrimp and Vegetable Stir-Fry

Preparation time = 25 minutes

Ingredients

- 1 lb (about 450g) Shrimp, peeled and deveined
- 2 cups Broccoli, cut into florets
- 1 Bell Pepper (any color), thinly sliced
- 1 cup Snap Peas, ends trimmed
- 1 tablespoon Olive or Vegetable Oil
- 2 tablespoons Low-Sodium Soy Sauce
- 1 tablespoon Freshly Grated Ginger

Servings = Serves 4

Mode of cooking: Stir-frying

Procedure:

Heat a tablespoon of oil in a wok or large skillet over medium-high heat. Add the shrimp and stir-fry for 2-3 minutes until they turn pink. Add the broccoli, bell peppers, and snap peas to the wok and continue stir-frying for an additional 3-4 minutes until the vegetables are tender-crisp. Season with a splash of low-sodium soy sauce and a sprinkle of freshly grated ginger.

Nutritional values: 228 calories | 25g protein | 9g fat | 14g carbohydrates

Recipe 3: Japanese-Inspired Miso Soup with Tofu and Scallions

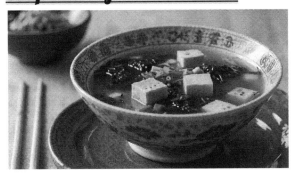

Preparation time = 15 minutes

Ingredients

- 4 cups Water
- 3 tablespoons Miso Paste
- 6 ounces Firm Tofu, cubed
- 2 tablespoons Wakame Seaweed, chopped
- 2 Scallions, finely sliced

Servings = Serves 2

Mode of cooking: Simmering

Procedure:

Bring 4 cups of water to a gentle simmer in a saucepan. Add 3 tablespoons of miso paste and stir until dissolved. Gently stir in 6 ounces of cubed firm tofu and 2 tablespoons of chopped wakame seaweed. Allow the soup to simmer for 5-7 minutes, then stir in 2 finely sliced scallions.

Nutritional values: 163 calories | 14g protein | 9g fat | 9g carbohydrates

Recipe 4: Soba Noodle Salad with Ginger Dressing

Preparation time = 30 minutes

Ingredients

- 8 ounces Soba Noodles
- 1 large Cucumber
- 2 medium Carrots
- 1 cup Shelled Edamane
- 2 tablespoons Grated Fresh Ginger
- 1/4 cup Rice Vinegar
- 1 tablespoon Toasted Sesame Oil

Servings = Serves 4

Mode of cooking: Boiling

Procedure:

Cook 8 ounces of soba noodles according to the package instructions, then rinse under cold water and drain well. In a large bowl, toss the cooked soba noodles with thinly sliced cucumbers, julienned carrots, and shelled edamame. Drizzle with a dressing made from grated fresh ginger, rice vinegar, and a touch of toasted sesame oil.

Nutritional values: 285 calories | 12g protein | 4g fat | 52g carbohydrates

Recipe 5: Thai Basil Chicken Lettuce Wraps

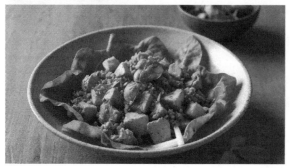

Preparation time = 25 minutes

Ingredients

- 1 pound Ground Chicken
- 1 cup Fresh Basil, coarsely chopped
- 1 cup Water Chestnuts, diced
- 1 tablespoon Low-Sodium Fish Sauce
- Lettuce Leaves (e.g., Butter, Romaine, or Iceberg) for serving

Servings = Serves 4

Mode of cooking: Pan-searing

Procedure:

In a skillet over medium heat, cook 1 pound of ground chicken until no longer pink. Stir in water chestnuts, chopped fresh basil, and a splash of low-sodium fish sauce. Simmer for 5-7 minutes until the flavors meld, then serve the chicken mixture in lettuce leaves.

Nutritional values: 198 calories | 23g protein | 8g fat | 6g carbohydrates

4.5.2 Mediterranean Delights: Heart-Healthy Fats and Grains

In this segment dedicated to Mediterranean-inspired dishes for individuals maintaining a diverticulitis-friendly diet, we bring you an assortment of recipes that are rich in heart-healthy fats and wholesome grains. From fiber-packed legumes to nutritious whole grains, these recipes encompass the essence of the Mediterranean diet while prioritizing ingredients conducive to digestive wellness.

Recipe 1: Greek-Style Baked Chicken with Lemon and Herbs

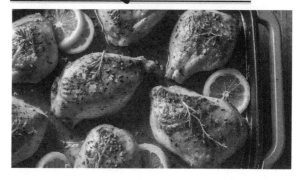

Preparation time = 30 minutes

Ingredients

- 4 Chicken Thighs (about 1.5 pounds)
- 2 Fresh Lemons
- 4 cloves Garlic, minced
- 2 teaspoons Dried Oregano
- Salt and Pepper, to taste

Servings = Serves 4

Mode of cooking: Baking

Procedure:

Preheat the oven to 375°F (190°C). Arrange the chicken thighs in a baking dish and season with minced garlic, dried oregano, and a generous squeeze of fresh lemon juice. Bake for 35-40 minutes or until the chicken is golden brown and thoroughly cooked.

Nutritional values: 279 calories | 27g protein | 17g fat | 4g carbohydrates

Recipe 2: Quinoa and Chickpea Salad with Cucumber and Feta

Preparation time = 25 minutes

Ingredients

- 1 cup Quinoa
- 2 cups Water
- 1 can (15 oz) Chickpeas, drained and rinsed
- 1 large Cucumber, diced
- 1 cup Feta Cheese, crumbled
- 3 tablespoons Extra Virgin Olive Oil
- Juice of 1 Lemon
- 2 tablespoons Fresh Parsley, chopped
- Salt and Pepper, to taste

Servings = Serves 4

Mode of cooking: Boiling

Procedure:

Rinse 1 cup of quinoa under running water, then cook in 2 cups of water until tender. Combine the cooked quinoa with canned chickpeas, diced cucumber, and crumbled feta cheese. Drizzle with a dressing made of extra virgin olive oil, lemon juice, and fresh chopped parsley.

Nutritional values: 289 calories | 12g protein | 12g fat | 36g carbohydrates

Recipe 3: Sicilian-Style Grilled Eggplant and Zucchini

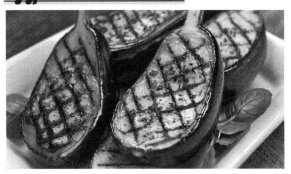

Preparation time = 20 minutes

Ingredients

- 1 medium Eggplant
- 2 Zucchinis
- 2 tablespoons Olive Oil
- 1 tablespoon Italian Herbs (blend of dried basil, oregano, rosemary, and thyme)
- Salt and Pepper, to taste

Servings = Serves 4

Mode of cooking: Grilling

Procedure:

Preheat a grill to medium-high heat. Slice 1 medium eggplant and 2 zucchinis into 1/2-inch thick rounds. Brush the vegetables with olive oil and sprinkle with Italian herbs, then grill for 3-4 minutes per side until tender.

Nutritional values: 132 calories | 4g protein | 7g fat | 16g carbohydrates

Recipe 4: Tuscan-Style White Bean and Tomato Soup

Preparation time = 35 minutes

Ingredients

- 2 cans (each 15 oz) Cannellini Beans, drained and rinsed
- 1 can (14.5 oz) Diced Tomatoes
- 4 cloves Garlic, minced
- 1 tablespoon Fresh Rosemary, finely chopped
- 2 tablespoons Olive Oil
- 4 cups Vegetable Broth
- Salt and Pepper, to taste
- Extra Virgin Olive Oil for drizzling

Servings = Serves 6

Mode of cooking: Simmering

Procedure:

In a large pot, heat olive oil and sauté minced garlic and fresh rosemary until fragrant. Stir in canned diced tomatoes and drained cannellini beans, then add vegetable broth and simmer for 20 minutes. Season with salt and pepper, and serve with a drizzle of extra virgin olive oil.

Nutritional values: 195 calories | 11g protein | 2g fat | 35g carbohydrates

Recipe 5: Moroccan-Inspired Couscous with Almonds and Dried Apricots

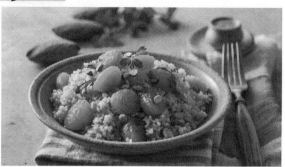

Preparation time = 20 minutes

Ingredients

- 1 cup Couscous
- 1/2 cup Slivered Almonds
- 1/2 cup Dried Apricots, diced
- 1 1/4 cups Water or Chicken/Vegetable Broth (for preparing couscous)
- Salt (optional and as per the couscous package instructions)
- 1 tablespoon Olive Oil or Butter (optional and as per the couscous package instructions)

Servings = Serves 4

Mode of cooking: Steaming

Procedure:

Prepare 1 cup of couscous according to package instructions. Fluff the cooked couscous with a fork and toss with slivered almonds and diced dried apricots. Serve as a flavorful and texturally diverse side dish.

Nutritional values: 281 calories | 8g protein | 7g fat | 49g carbohydrates

4.5.3 Latin American Fare: Mild Yet Robust Flavor Profiles

In this segment showcasing Latin American-inspired dishes for individuals on a diverticulitis-friendly diet, we present you with an array of flavorful and nutrient-dense recipes. By incorporating mild spices and bold aromatic herbs, these dishes honor the vibrant culinary traditions of the region while prioritizing ingredients conducive to digestive health.

Recipe 1: Cuban-Style Roasted Pork Tenderloin

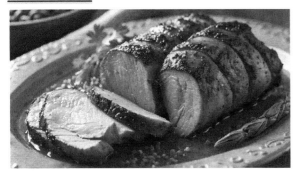

Preparation time = 45 minutes

Ingredients

- 1 lb. Pork Tenderloin
- 4 cloves Garlic, minced
- 1 tablespoon Ground Cumin
- 1/4 teaspoon Cayenne Pepper (adjust to taste)
- Salt to taste
- 2 tablespoons Olive Oil (optional, for a richer rub)

Servings = Serves 4

Mode of cooking: Roasting

Procedure:

Preheat the oven to 375°F (190°C). Rub a 1-lb. pork tenderloin with a mixture of minced garlic, ground cumin, and a pinch of cayenne pepper. Roast for 30-35 minutes or until the internal temperature reaches 145°F (63°C).

Nutritional values: 156 calories | 24g protein | 5g fat | 1g carbohydrates

Recipe 2: Vegetarian Black Bean and Sweet Potato Chili

Preparation time = 35 minutes

Ingredients

- 2 large Sweet Potatoes, peeled and diced
- 2 cans (15 oz each) Black Beans, drained and rinsed
- 1 can (14.5 oz) Diced Tomatoes
- 1 tablespoon Ground Cumin
- 1 tablespoon Chili Powder
- Salt to taste
- 2 tablespoons Olive Oil
- Optional: Plain Greek Yogurt for serving

Servings = Serves 6

Mode of cooking: Stovetop

Procedure:

In a large pot, sauté diced sweet potatoes until tender, then add drained and rinsed canned black beans, diced tomatoes, and a mixture of cumin and chili powder. Simmer for 20-25 minutes or until the chili has thickened and the flavors have melded. Serve with a dollop of plain Greek yogurt for added creaminess.

Nutritional values: 190 calories | 10g protein | 1g fat | 11g carbohydrates

---

Recipe 3: Peruvian-Style Ceviche with Avocado and Sweet Potato

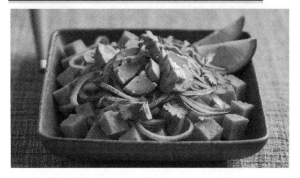

Preparation time = 30 minutes

Ingredients:

- 1 lb. White Fish (such as sea bass, tilapia, or cod), cut into bite-sized pieces
- 1 cup Fresh Lime Juice (from approximately 8-10 limes)
- 1 medium Red Onion, finely minced
- 1 large Sweet Potato, cooked and diced
- 1 large Avocado, sliced
- Salt to taste
- Optional garnishes: Cilantro, chili pepper slices

Servings = Serves 4

Mode of cooking: Citric acid "cooking"

Procedure:

Cut 1 lb. of white fish into bite-sized pieces, and marinate in a mixture of fresh lime juice and minced red onion for 15-20 minutes. Arrange cooked diced sweet potato and sliced avocado on a plate, and top with the ceviche mixture.

Nutritional values: 228 calories | 23g protein | 11g fat | 12g carbohydrates

---

Recipe 4: Brazilian-Style Collard Greens with Garlic and Lemon

Preparation time = 20 minutes

Ingredients

- 1 bunch Collard Greens (approximately 10-12 large leaves)
- 3 tablespoons Olive Oil
- 4 cloves Garlic, minced
- 1 Lemon, juiced
- Salt, to taste

Servings = Serves 4

Mode of cooking: Sauteing

Procedure:

Wash and destem 1 bunch of collard greens, then chiffonade the leaves. In a sauté pan, heat olive oil and minced garlic until fragrant, then add the collard greens and sauté until wilted. Finish with a squeeze of fresh lemon juice and a pinch of salt.

Nutritional values: 47 calories | 2g protein | 3g fat | 5g carbohydrates

Recipe 5: Mexican-Style Spiced Sweet Potato and Black Bean Salad

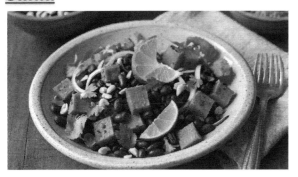

Preparation time = 25 minutes

Ingredients

- 2 large Sweet Potatoes, peeled and cubed (about 4 cups)
- 1 tablespoon Olive Oil
- 1 teaspoon Ground Cumin
- 1 teaspoon Smoked Paprika
- 1 can (15 oz) Black Beans, drained and rinsed
- 2 tablespoons Fresh Lime Juice (approximately juice of 1 lime)
- Salt to taste
- ¼ cup Toasted Pepitas (pumpkin seeds) for garnish
- ¼ cup Crumbled Cotija Cheese for garnish

Servings = Serves 4

Mode of cooking: Roasting

Procedure:

Roast cubed sweet potato until tender, then toss with drained and rinsed canned black beans, cumin, smoked paprika, and a squeeze of fresh lime juice. Serve the salad chilled or at room temperature, alongside toasted pepitas and crumbled cotija cheese.

Nutritional values: 201 calories | 8g protein | 3g fat | 37g carbohydrates

These Latin American-inspired recipes marry the health-enhancing benefits of dietary fiber and wholesome whole foods with the evocative aromas and flavors of the region. Enjoy the best of both worlds, and savor every bite with pleasure and gratitude.

4.5.4 European Classics: Comforting Meals Reimagined for Gut Health

In this segment highlighting European classic dishes adapted for individuals with diverticulitis, we present a selection of comforting and nutritious recipes that honor the culinary traditions of the region while prioritizing ingredients that support gut health.

Recipe 1: Italian-Inspired Chicken and Vegetable Sheet Pan Dinner

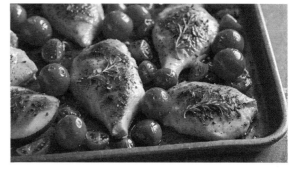

Preparation time = 40 minutes

Ingredients :

- 4 Chicken Breasts, thinly sliced (about 1.5 lbs or 680 grams)
- 2 medium Zucchinis, diced (about 2 cups)
- 2 cups Cherry Tomatoes, halved
- 2 tablespoons Italian Seasoning
- 2 tablespoons Olive Oil
- Salt and Pepper to taste

Servings = Serves 4

Mode of cooking: Roasting

Procedure:

Preheat the oven to 400°F (200°C). Place thinly sliced chicken breast, diced zucchini, and halved cherry tomatoes on a sheet pan, then season with Italian seasoning and a drizzle of olive oil. Roast for 20-25 minutes or until the chicken is cooked through and the vegetables are tender.

Nutritional values: 235 calories | 27g protein | 6g fat | 18g carbohydrates

Recipe 2: French-Style Lentil Salad with Dijon Vinaigrette

Preparation time = 30 minutes

Ingredients

- 1 cup Green Lentils
- 2 medium Carrots, diced (about 1 cup)
- 1 Red Bell Pepper, chopped (about 1 cup)
- 1 tablespoon Dijon Mustard
- 3 tablespoons Olive Oil
- 1 tablespoon Red Wine Vinegar
- Salt and Pepper to taste

Servings = Serves 4

Mode of cooking: Stovetop

Procedure:

Cook green lentils according to package instructions until al dente, then drain and let cool. Toss the lentils with diced carrots, chopped red bell pepper, and a homemade vinaigrette made with Dijon mustard, olive oil, and red wine vinegar. Chill the salad before serving.

Nutritional values: 182 calories | 10g protein | 4g fat | 28g carbohydrates

Recipe 3: Spanish-Inspired Garlic Shrimp with Lemon and Parsley

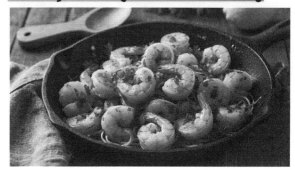

Preparation time = 20 minutes

Ingredients

- 1 pound (approx. 450 grams) Shrimp, peeled and deveined
- 4 cloves Garlic, minced
- Juice of 1 Lemon
- 1/4 cup Parsley, finely chopped
- 2 tablespoons Olive Oil
- Salt and Pepper to taste

Servings = Serves 4

Mode of cooking: Sauteing

Procedure:

In a large skillet, sauté peeled shrimp with minced garlic until the shrimp turn pink and opaque. Squeeze fresh lemon juice over the shrimp, then garnish with chopped parsley before serving.

Nutritional values: 159 calories | 24g protein | 6g fat | 2g carbohydrates

Recipe 4: English-Style Mashed Potatoes with Chives

Preparation time = 35 minutes

Ingredients

- 2 pounds (approx. 900 grams) Potatoes
- 1/4 cup Chives, finely chopped
- 2 tablespoons Olive Oil
- Salt and Pepper to taste

Servings = Serves 4

Mode of cooking: Boiling and Mashing

Procedure:

Peel and dice potatoes, then boil until tender. Drain well. Mash the potatoes with a splash of olive oil and finely chopped chives until smooth and creamy.

Nutritional values: 162 calories | 3g protein | 4g fat | 30g carbohydrates

Recipe 5: Greek-Inspired Grilled Lemon Herb Chicken Skewers

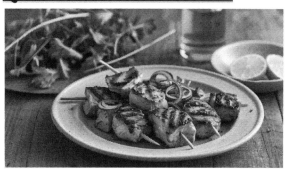

Preparation time = 30 minutes

Ingredients

- 1.5 pounds (approx. 680 grams) boneless Chicken Thighs
- Zest of 1 Lemon
- 2 tablespoons dried Oregano
- 2 tablespoons Olive Oil
- 1 large Red Onion, cut into chunks
- Salt and Pepper to taste

Servings = Serves 4

Mode of cooking: Grilling

Procedure:

Cut boneless chicken thighs into chunks and marinate in a mixture of lemon zest, dried oregano, and olive oil for 15-20 minutes. Thread the marinated chicken onto skewers with red onion slices and grill until cooked through.

Nutritional values: 198 calories | 24g protein | 10g fat | 3g carbohydrates

4.5.5 Middle Eastern Dishes: Spiced Options for a Diverse Palate

In this section featuring Middle Eastern-inspired dishes tailored for individuals following a diverticulitis-friendly diet, we present a collection of flavorful and spiced recipes that pay homage to the rich and diverse culinary heritage of the region. Each dish incorporates ingredients that align with the dietary guidelines for digestive health, ensuring a delightful and nourishing dining experience.

Recipe 1: Moroccan-Inspired Chicken Tagine with Apricots and Almonds

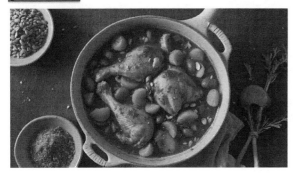

Preparation time = 50 minutes

Ingredients

- 1.5 pounds (approx. 680 grams) Chicken Thighs, skin-on
- 1 cup (approx. 140 grams) Dried Apricots, diced
- 1/2 cup (approx. 70 grams) Whole Almonds
- 2 tablespoons Ras el Hanout spice blend
- Salt and Pepper to taste
- 2 tablespoons Olive Oil

Servings = Serves 4

Mode of cooking: Stovetop

Procedure:

In a tagine or heavy-bottomed pot, brown skin-on chicken thighs, then add diced dried apricots, whole almonds, and a sprinkle of Ras el Hanout spice blend. Cover and simmer gently for 30-35 minutes until the chicken is tender and the flavors have melded.

Nutritional values: 287 calories | 30g protein | 15g fat | 11g carbohydrates

---

Recipe 2: Lebanese-Style Tabbouleh Salad with Quinoa

Preparation time = 20 minutes

Ingredients

- 1 cup (approx. 170 grams) Quinoa
- 2 cups (approx. 60 grams) fresh Parsley, finely chopped
- 2 medium Tomatoes, diced
- 1 large Cucumber, diced
- 3 tablespoons Extra Virgin Olive Oil
- Juice of 1 Lemon
- Salt to taste

Servings = Serves 4

Mode of cooking: Steaming and Chopping

Procedure:

Cook quinoa according to package instructions, then let cool. Mix the cooked quinoa with finely chopped parsley, diced tomatoes, and diced cucumber, then dress with extra virgin olive oil and lemon juice.

Nutritional values: 192 calories | 5g protein | 7g fat | 28g carbohydrates

Recipe 3: Turkish-Style Yogurt and Cucumber Soup (Cacik)

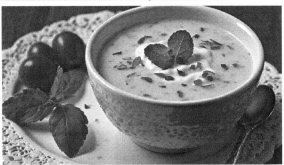

Preparation time = 15 minutes

Ingredients

- 2 cups (approx. 475 grams) Greek Yogurt
- 1 large Cucumber
- 1 clove Garlic, minced
- 2 tablespoons fresh Mint, finely chopped
- Salt to taste

Servings = Serves 4

Mode of cooking: No-Cook

Procedure:

Grate and squeeze excess moisture from a cucumber, then combine with Greek yogurt, minced garlic, and chopped mint. Chill the soup for at least 1 hour before serving.

Nutritional values: 78 calories | 8g protein | 2g fat | 7g carbohydrates

Recipe 4: Persian-Inspired Grilled Beef Kebabs with Sumac and Turmeric

Preparation time = 35 minutes

Ingredients

- 1 lb (approx. 450 grams) Beef Sirloin
- 1 large Onion
- 2 teaspoons Sumac
- 1 teaspoon Turmeric
- 3 tablespoons Olive Oil
- Salt and freshly ground Black Pepper, to taste

Servings = Serves 4

Mode of cooking: Grilling

Procedure:

Cube beef sirloin and marinate with thinly sliced onion, sumac, turmeric, and olive oil for 20-25 minutes. Thread the marinated beef onto skewers and grill to desired doneness.

Nutritional values: 251 calories | 27g protein | 15g fat | 3g carbohydrates

Recipe 5: Israeli-Inspired Eggplant and Tomato Shakshuka

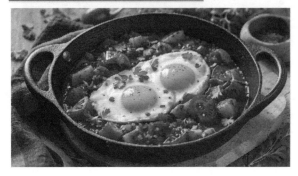

Preparation time = 40 minutes

Ingredients

- 2 medium-sized Eggplants
- 4 large Tomatoes
- 1 large Bell Pepper (any color)
- 1 teaspoon Ground Cumin
- 1 teaspoon Paprika (optional for added flavor and color)
- 1 small Onion, finely chopped
- 2 cloves Garlic, minced
- 4 large Eggs
- 2 tablespoons Olive Oil
- Salt and Pepper, to taste
- Fresh Parsley for garnish (optional)

Servings = Serves 4

Mode of cooking: Stovetop

Procedure:

Sauté diced eggplant, tomatoes, and bell pepper in a skillet until softened, then season with ground cumin and other desired spices. Create wells in the vegetable mixture and crack eggs into the wells. Cover and cook until the eggs are set to your preference.

Nutritional values: 168 calories | 8g protein | 8g fat | 18g carbohydrates

Chapter 5: Meal Planning and Preparation

5.1 Creating a Diverticulitis Meal Plan: A Week's Worth of Ideas

As someone navigating the complexities of diverticulitis, designing a well-thought-out meal plan is crucial for managing your condition effectively and minimizing discomfort. This comprehensive guide aims to provide you with practical insights and inspiration for crafting a week's worth of nutritious, gut-friendly meals tailored to support your digestive health.

Understanding Your Dietary Needs

When planning your diverticulitis meal plan, it's essential to focus on including high-fiber foods to promote regular bowel movements and maintain gut health.

However, it's equally important to avoid trigger foods that can exacerbate inflammation and contribute to flare-ups. Incorporating a variety of nutrients, such as lean proteins, healthy fats, whole grains, and low-fiber fruits and vegetables, can help create a balanced and sustainable eating pattern.

Day 1: Kick-Start Your Week

Begin your week with a nourishing breakfast of Greek yogurt topped with fresh berries and a sprinkle of chia seeds. For lunch, prepare a quinoa salad with roasted vegetables and grilled chicken, drizzled with a lemon vinaigrette. In the evening, enjoy a comforting meal of baked salmon with asparagus and wild rice pilaf.

Day 2: Midweek Boost

For a hearty breakfast, indulge in an omelet stuffed with spinach, tomatoes, and feta cheese. Lunch can consist of a colorful spinach and strawberry salad with grilled shrimp and a balsamic glaze. Cap off your day with a cozy bowl of lentil soup paired with a side of whole grain bread.

Day 3: Variety Is Key

Start your day with a nutrient-packed smoothie made with spinach, banana, almond milk, and a scoop of protein powder. Settle into lunch with a turkey and avocado wrap on a whole wheat tortilla, accompanied by a side of crudites. For dinner, savor a vegetable stir-fry with tofu and brown rice, seasoned with ginger and garlic.

Day 4: Savory Delights

Kick off your morning with a bowl of oatmeal topped with sliced almonds and honey. At midday, relish a caprese salad with fresh mozzarella, tomatoes, and basil, drizzled with olive oil and balsamic vinegar. End your day with a comforting chicken and vegetable curry served with fluffy basmati rice.

Day 5: Fresh and Flavorful

Enjoy a refreshing breakfast of overnight oats with diced apples, cinnamon, and a dollop of almond butter. For lunch, whip up a tuna salad with mixed greens and a lemon-dill dressing. Wind down with a zesty shrimp and vegetable skewers served with quinoa and a squeeze of fresh lemon.

Day 6: Simple Pleasures

Start your day with a protein-packed smoothie bowl topped with granola and sliced bananas. Lunch can feature a Greek-inspired salad with cucumbers, olives, and feta cheese drizzled with a homemade tzatziki dressing. Indulge in a comforting dinner of baked cod with roasted Brussels sprouts and sweet potatoes.

Day 7: Satisfying End to the Week

Round off your week with a leisurely brunch of whole grain pancakes topped with mixed berries and a dollop of Greek yogurt. For a light lunch, relish a beet and goat cheese salad with a citrus vinaigrette. Conclude your week on a high note with a hearty beef and vegetable stew simmered to perfection.

Crafting a diverse and nutritious meal plan for diverticulitis management doesn't have to be daunting. By incorporating a wide range of wholesome ingredients, planning balanced meals, and listening to your body's cues, you can navigate your dietary journey with confidence and comfort. Embrace this week's worth of meal ideas as a foundation for your culinary exploration and digestive well-being.

5.2 Meal Prep Strategies for Busy Lifestyles

Incorporating a nutritious and gut-friendly diet into a fast-paced lifestyle can be challenging, especially when managing a condition like diverticulitis. However, with strategic meal planning and preparation, even the busiest individuals can stay on track with their dietary needs. Here, we delve into essential meal prep strategies tailored for those navigating hectic schedules while prioritizing their digestive health.

Simplify Your Ingredients

When it comes to meal prep, simplicity is key. Opt for whole, minimally processed ingredients that are gentle on your digestive system. Incorporate a variety of lean proteins, such as chicken, fish, and tofu, alongside vibrant fruits and vegetables like leafy greens, berries, and squash. By keeping your ingredient list straightforward, you can streamline your meal prep process and ensure your dishes are both flavorful and nutritious.

Batch Cooking for Efficiency

Batch cooking is a game-changer for individuals with busy lifestyles. Dedicate a few hours each week to prepare large batches of staple foods like whole grains, roasted vegetables, and protein sources. Portion out these components into convenient containers, allowing you to assemble quick and balanced meals throughout the week. This approach not only saves time but also helps you stay consistent with your dietary goals.

Strategic Snack Planning

Snacks play a crucial role in maintaining energy levels and preventing overeating during busy days. Prepare nutritious snack options in advance, such as raw nuts, Greek yogurt with honey, or hummus with vegetable sticks. Portion out these snacks into grab-and-go containers or bags, so you always have a healthy option on hand when hunger strikes. Planning your snacks ahead of time can help you avoid reaching for less optimal choices when pressed for time.

Embrace Make-Ahead Meals

Make-ahead meals are a lifesaver for individuals seeking convenience without compromising on nutrition. Choose recipes that can be prepared in advance, such as casseroles, soups, and salads. Invest time in cooking a large batch of these dishes over the weekend, portioning them into individual servings that can be easily reheated or enjoyed cold throughout the week. Make-ahead meals ensure that you always have a wholesome option available, even on the busiest of days.

Utilize Time-Saving Kitchen Tools

Efficiency in meal prep often comes down to the tools you use in the kitchen. Invest in time-saving appliances like a slow cooker, pressure cooker, or food processor to streamline your cooking process. These tools can help you prepare meals more efficiently, allowing you to enjoy nutritious and flavorful dishes without spending hours in the kitchen. By embracing modern kitchen gadgets, you can make meal prep both convenient and enjoyable.

Customize Your Meal Prep Routine

Every individual has unique dietary preferences and requirements, so it's essential to tailor your meal prep routine to suit your specific needs. Experiment with different recipes, flavors, and cooking methods to discover what works best for you. Listen to your body's cues and adjust your meal prep strategy accordingly to ensure that you're nourishing yourself in a way that aligns with your digestive health goals.

Incorporating these practical meal prep strategies into your routine can help you navigate your busy lifestyle while prioritizing your digestive health. By simplifying your ingredients, embracing batch cooking, strategically planning snacks, preparing make-ahead meals, utilizing time-saving kitchen tools, and customizing your approach, you can establish a sustainable meal prep routine that supports your overall well-being.

5.3 Shopping and Ingredient Swaps: Navigating the Grocery Store

Embarking on a journey towards managing diverticulitis through dietary adjustments involves a crucial aspect: navigating the grocery store with confidence and making informed ingredient swaps that support your digestive health goals. By understanding which foods to prioritize and which to avoid, you can empower yourself to shop strategically and select gut-friendly ingredients that will serve as the foundation for your meals.

Understanding Your Grocery Store Environment

As you step into the aisles of your local grocery store, it's essential to approach your shopping experience with a mindset centered on your health and well-being. Familiarize yourself with the layout of the store and identify key sections that align with your dietary needs. Focus on the perimeter of the store, where fresh produce, lean proteins, and whole grains are typically located. By prioritizing these sections, you can fill your cart with nutrient-dense ingredients that form the basis of a gut-friendly diet.

Embracing Fresh, Wholesome Ingredients

When selecting ingredients for your meals, opt for fresh, whole foods that are minimally processed and free from artificial additives. Incorporating a variety of colorful fruits and vegetables not only enhances the visual appeal of your dishes but also provides essential vitamins, minerals, and fiber to support your digestive system. Choose lean sources of protein such as poultry, fish, and plant-based alternatives like legumes and tofu to promote satiety and muscle health while reducing the strain on your digestive tract.

Making Smart Ingredient Swaps

Navigating the grocery store can be overwhelming, especially when faced with a multitude of food choices. Making smart ingredient swaps can help you tailor your meals to support your diverticulitis management while still enjoying delicious and satisfying dishes. Consider swapping out high-fiber foods that may be trigger foods for your condition with lower-fiber alternatives. For example, if whole grains like wheat cause discomfort, explore gluten-free options such as rice, quinoa, or oats to provide nutritious alternatives without compromising on taste or texture.

Reading Labels and Making Informed Choices

As you scan the shelves for ingredients to incorporate into your meals, take the time to read labels carefully and familiarize yourself with common terms related to food packaging. Look for products that are low in added sugars, sodium, and artificial preservatives to minimize potential triggers for diverticulitis flare-ups. Opt for whole foods whenever possible and prioritize ingredients with recognizable names and minimal processing to ensure that you are nourishing your body with foods that support your digestive health.

Building a Diverse and Balanced Pantry

Stocking your pantry with a diverse array of ingredients lays the foundation for creating a wide range of flavorful and gut-friendly meals. Ensure that your pantry includes staples such as olive oil, herbs and spices, canned beans, and low-sodium broths to enhance the taste and nutritional value of your dishes. Experiment with different ingredients to add variety to your meals while keeping a balance between high-fiber and low-fiber options based on your individual needs and tolerance levels.

Seeking Guidance from Health Professionals

Navigating the grocery store and making ingredient swaps can be a learning process, especially when managing a complex condition like diverticulitis. Don't hesitate to seek guidance from registered dietitians for healthcare professionals who can offer personalized recommendations tailored to your specific dietary requirements. By collaborating with experts in the field of digestive health, you can gain invaluable insights and confidence in selecting ingredients that support your overall well-being.

Chapter 6: Lifestyle Modification and Additional Tips

6.1 Exercise and Diverticulitis: What You Need to Know

Physical activity plays a crucial role in managing diverticulitis and promoting overall health and well-being. Engaging in regular exercise can help alleviate symptoms, reduce the risk of diverticulitis flare-ups, and improve the quality of life for individuals dealing with this condition. In this section, we will explore the relationship between exercise and diverticulitis, providing you with essential information and practical tips to incorporate physical activity into your daily routine.

The Benefits of Exercise for Diverticulitis Management

Exercise offers a multitude of benefits for individuals managing diverticulitis. By staying physically active, you can improve bowel regularity and promote healthy digestion. Regular exercise helps regulate intestinal contractions, reducing the likelihood of bowel spasms and constipation, which are common triggers for diverticulitis flare-ups.

Additionally, exercise can aid in maintaining a healthy weight, which is vital for overall well-being and diverticulitis management. Shedding excess pounds can help alleviate strain on the intestine, minimizing pressure and reducing the risk of developing diverticula, or pouches in the colon wall, which can become inflamed and cause diverticulitis.

Exercise also offers significant benefits for maintaining cardiovascular health, strengthening muscles, and boosting immunity. When you engage in physical activity, blood circulation improves, allowing essential nutrients and oxygen to reach the colon and other organs, contributing to overall gut health.

Choosing the Right Exercise for Diverticulitis

When selecting exercise activities, it's essential to opt for low-impact and low-intensity exercises, especially during flare-ups or when symptoms are present. High-impact activities or exercises that involve intense abdominal contractions, such as heavy weightlifting or vigorous sit-ups, may aggravate diverticulitis symptoms and should be avoided during these times.

Instead, consider incorporating exercises such as walking, swimming, cycling, or gentle yoga into your fitness routine. These activities provide gentle movement that promotes blood flow and helps alleviate symptoms without putting excessive strain on the digestive system. Always listen to your body and adjust the intensity and duration of workouts based on your comfort level and any guidance provided by your healthcare professional.

Tips for Incorporating Exercise into your Routine

Making exercise a regular part of your daily routine is crucial for effective diverticulitis management. Follow these practical tips for incorporating exercise into your lifestyle:

- **Start Slowly**: If you have been inactive or are new to exercise, start with low-intensity activities and gradually increase duration and intensity over time. This approach allows your body to adjust and adapt, reducing the risk of triggering symptoms.
- **Find Activities You Enjoy**: Engaging in exercises that you genuinely enjoy increases the likelihood of sticking with your routine. Whether it's dancing, gardening, or joining a recreational sports team, choose activities that bring you joy and keep you motivated.
- **Make it a Habit**: Aim for at least 30 minutes of exercise most days of the week. Schedule dedicated time for physical activity, just as you would for any other important task. Consistency is key to reaping the long-term benefits of exercise.
- **Mix it Up:** Vary your exercise routine to prevent boredom and work different muscle groups. Consider alternating between cardiovascular activities, strength training, and flexibility exercises to achieve a well-rounded fitness routine.
- **Listen to Your Body**: Pay attention to how your body responds to exercise. If you experience any discomfort or notice an increase in symptoms, modify or reduce the intensity of your workouts. It's essential to strike a balance between challenging yourself and avoiding exacerbation of diverticulitis symptoms.
- **Stay Hydrated**: Remember to drink sufficient amounts of water before, during, and after exercise. Staying hydrated helps maintain proper digestion and alleviates the risk of dehydration, which can worsen constipation and other diverticulitis symptoms.
- **Seek Professional Guidance**: If you have any concerns or specific limitations, consult a healthcare professional or a qualified fitness instructor who can provide personalized guidance based on your unique needs and condition.

Incorporating exercise into your diverticulitis management plan is a powerful way to support your overall health and well-being. Engaging in regular physical activity can alleviate symptoms, reduce the risk of flare-ups, and enhance your quality of life. Remember to choose low-impact exercises, start slowly, find activities you enjoy, and make exercise a habit.

6.2 The Mind-Gut Connection: Understanding How Stress Affects Symptoms

Stress is an inevitable part of our lives, and it can have a significant impact on our overall well-being, including our digestive health. For individuals dealing with diverticulitis, stress can potentially worsen symptoms and trigger painful flare-ups. In this section, we will explore the mind-gut connection and help you understand how stress affects diverticulitis symptoms. By gaining this understanding, you can take proactive steps to manage stress and maintain control over your health.

The Mind-Gut Connection: Explained

The mind-gut connection refers to the intricate relationship between our brain and our digestive system. The two are connected by an extensive network of nerves and chemicals, allowing them to communicate and influence one another. This connection is bidirectional, meaning that both the brain and the gut can send signals to each other, affecting various functions.

When we experience stress, our body goes into the "fight or flight" mode, releasing stress hormones such as cortisol and adrenaline. These hormones can have a direct impact on our gastrointestinal system, causing certain changes in our digestive function. For individuals with diverticulitis, stress can disrupt the delicate balance within the gut, leading to increased inflammation, altered gut motility, and heightened sensitivity to pain.

How Stress Affects Diverticulitis Symptoms

Stress can exacerbate diverticulitis symptoms by triggering inflammation and aggravating the existing inflammation in the colon. When we are under stress, our body's immune response can become dysregulated, leading to an overactive inflammatory response in the gut. This increased inflammation can worsen the symptoms of diverticulitis, including abdominal pain, bloating, constipation, and diarrhea.

Moreover, stress can also affect the motility of the intestines, leading to irregular bowel movements. Some individuals may experience increased contractions, resulting in diarrhea, while others may have reduced contractions, leading to constipation. These changes in bowel movements can further exacerbate diverticulitis symptoms and increase the risk of flare-ups.

It is crucial to note that while stress can exacerbate symptoms, it does not directly cause diverticulitis. Diverticulitis is primarily caused by the formation of diverticula, small pouches that develop in the colon wall. However, managing stress and reducing its impact on your gut can significantly improve your overall well-being and the management of diverticulitis symptoms.

Stress Management Techniques for Diverticulitis

Managing stress is vital for individuals with diverticulitis to minimize the impact of stress on their symptoms and overall gut health. Here are some stress management techniques you can incorporate into your daily routine:

- **Relaxation Techniques**: Engage in relaxation techniques, such as deep breathing exercises, progressive muscle relaxation, or guided meditation. These techniques promote relaxation, reduce stress levels, and help calm the mind and body.
- **Regular Exercise**: Physical activity is not only beneficial for diverticulitis management but also an excellent stress-buster. Engaging in regular exercise, such as walking, swimming, or yoga, can help reduce stress hormone levels and promote a sense of well-being.
- **Prioritize Self-Care:** Dedicate time each day for activities that bring you joy and help you relax. This can include hobbies, reading, spending time in nature, or enjoying a hot bath. Prioritizing self-care is essential for stress management.
- **Stress-Relieving Activities:** Engage in activities that help relieve stress and promote relaxation. This can vary from person to person and may include activities such as listening to soothing music, practicing mindfulness, journaling, or engaging in creative pursuits.
- **Support Network:** Seek support from friends, family, or a support group. Talking and sharing your feelings with others who understand your experience can help reduce stress and create a sense of belonging.
- **Healthy Lifestyle Choices:** Maintain a healthy lifestyle by eating a balanced diet, getting enough restful sleep, and limiting the consumption of caffeine and alcohol. These lifestyle choices can contribute to better stress management and overall well-being.
- **Professional Support:** If stress becomes overwhelming or persists despite your efforts, do not hesitate to seek professional help. A mental health professional can provide guidance, support, and additional strategies to manage stress effectively.

Understanding the mind-gut connection and how stress affects diverticulitis symptoms is essential for taking control of your health and well-being. By managing stress, you can minimize its impact on your gut and promote a healthier digestive system. Incorporate stress management techniques into your daily routine, such as relaxation techniques, regular exercise, self-care activities, and seeking support when needed. Remember that stress management is a crucial component of diverticulitis management, allowing you to lead a balanced, enjoyable life while maintaining control over your condition.

6.3 Building Your Support System: Family, Friends, and Online Communities

As a passionate advocate for individuals navigating the complexities of diverticulitis, I understand the crucial role that a strong support system plays in effectively managing this condition. In the journey towards optimal health, building a reliable support network can provide invaluable emotional and practical assistance. Whether you've recently been diagnosed with diverticulitis or have been grappling with its challenges for some time, the assistance of family, friends, and online communities can enhance your ability to navigate this condition with confidence and empowerment.

The Power of Familial Support

At the heart of every individual's journey with diverticulitis lies the unwavering support of family members. Your loved ones are a source of compassion, understanding, and encouragement, making the burden of managing diverticulitis easier to bear. When it comes to dietary modifications, family members can embrace and reinforce your dietary adjustments, creating an environment conducive to your well-being. Their understanding and willingness to accommodate your dietary needs can alleviate the stress and anxiety associated with meal preparation and social gatherings, fostering a sense of inclusion and solidarity.

Embracing Supportive friendships

Beyond the confines of familial bonds, friends who offer unwavering support play a pivotal role in your journey with diverticulitis. Whether it's through offering a listening ear, accompanying you on leisurely walks, or simply being a reliable presence, true friends can provide solace and understanding. Cultivating open communication with friends and enlightening them about your dietary requirements can help them navigate social settings with sensitivity, facilitating an inclusive and supportive environment for your well-being.

The Benefits of Online Communities

In today's interconnected world, the power of online communities cannot be overstated. Engaging with virtual communities dedicated to diverticulitis allows you to connect with individuals who share similar experiences, challenges, and victories. These online platforms serve as a hub of shared knowledge, encouragement, and empathy. By participating in these communities, you can gain insights into real-life experiences, discover practical tips for symptom management, and access firsthand accounts of navigating dietary choices. Furthermore, the ability to seek advice, share concerns, and celebrate successes in a non-judgmental space can be profoundly uplifting and empowering.

Nurturing Your Support Network

Building and nurturing your support system, be it through familial bonds, friendships, or online communities, is a dynamic and ongoing process. Effective communication is the bedrock of these relationships, allowing you to express your needs, share your experiences, and seek understanding. It's essential to openly communicate your dietary requirements and the impact of diverticulitis on your daily life, empowering your support network to provide tailored assistance. By fostering understanding and collaboration within your support system, you can navigate the challenges of diverticulitis with resilience, assurance, and a sense of belonging.

Empowerment through Collective Strength

In the realm of diverticulitis management, the significance of a reliable support system extends far beyond emotional sustenance. Your support network can contribute to the practical aspects of your well-being, such as enabling you to adhere to dietary modifications, encouraging physical activity, and offering reassurance during moments of uncertainty. Embracing the collective strength of your support system empowers you to take charge of your health with confidence, alleviating the anxiety of making dietary choices and fostering a sense of control over your well-being.

The journey with diverticulitis is inherently enriched by the unwavering support of family, friends, and the broader community. As you navigate the intricacies of this condition, remember that you are not alone. Embrace the compassion and understanding of your loved ones, nurture your friendships, and seek solace, knowledge, and inspiration within online communities. By cultivating and cherishing your support system, you can approach the management of diverticulitis with resilience, empowerment, and a profound sense of unity. Let the collective strength of your support network serve as a beacon of hope and encouragement, guiding you towards a life of balance, fulfillment, and well-being.

Conclusion

In the dynamic realm of diverticulitis management, achieving a harmonious balance between dietary choices, symptom alleviation, and overall well-being is paramount. By embarking on this comprehensive culinary journey towards optimal health, you have taken a crucial step towards reclaiming control over your dietary decisions and ensuring a fulfilling, symptom-free lifestyle.

The Power of Knowledge and Confidence

Armed with a wealth of credible, up-to-date information on diverticulitis management, you are well-equipped to navigate the intricacies of this condition with confidence and assurance. By understanding the impact of different food choices on your digestive system, you can make informed decisions that promote digestive health and prevent painful flare-ups. Embrace the knowledge at your fingertips as a beacon of empowerment, guiding you towards a path of conscious food selection and symptom management.

Navigating Dietary Choices with Precision

As you embark on this culinary expedition, precision and mindfulness in your dietary choices are key to achieving optimal well-being. By incorporating a range of safe, nutritious ingredients tailored to your stage of diverticulitis, you can curate a diverse, flavorful menu that supports digestive health and minimizes discomfort. Embrace the art of ingredient selection as a powerful tool in crafting meals that nourish both body and soul, offering a delightful culinary experience without compromising your health goals.

Harmonizing Flavors and Textures

In the realm of diverticulitis-friendly cooking, the interplay of flavors and textures holds immense potential for creating satisfying, enjoyable meals that cater to your dietary needs. Embrace the harmonious fusion of ingredients to elevate your culinary creations, infusing each dish with a symphony of tastes and sensations. By experimenting with a diverse palette of flavors and textures, you can revel in the culinary artistry of diverticulitis management, savoring each meal as a delightful symphony of nourishment and pleasure.

Embracing Culinary Creativity

As you delve into the realm of diverticulitis-conscious cooking, unleash your culinary creativity to unveil a treasure trove of delectable, healthful recipes that cater to your specific dietary requirements. Infuse each dish with a personalized touch, incorporating your favorite ingredients and culinary preferences to craft meals that not only support your digestive health but also tantalize your taste buds. Embrace the joy of culinary experimentation as a gateway to discovering new flavors, textures, and culinary delights that enrich your dining experience and invigorate your well-being.

Savoring the Journey Ahead

With a trusted culinary companion by your side, you can embark on a journey towards digestive wellness that is both enriching and rewarding. Through the artful curation of diverticulitis-conscious recipes, you can savor each meal as a celebration of health, vitality, and culinary creativity. Embrace the evolution of your dietary journey with an open heart and a curious palate, relishing the flavors, aromas, and textures that define each gastronomic adventure. By savoring the culinary delights that lie ahead, you can transform your dietary choices into a source of nourishment, joy, and empowerment that fuels your path towards optimal well-being.

Empowerment Through Culinary Mastery

In the tapestry of diverticulitis management, culinary mastery emerges as a powerful tool for empowerment and self-care. By honing your culinary skills and embracing the art of diverticulitis-conscious cooking, you can cultivate a profound sense of agency and control over your dietary choices. Take pride in the culinary creations you craft, reveling in the virtuosity of each dish as a testament to your commitment to health and well-being. Through the mastery of diverticulitis-friendly cooking, you can empower yourself to take charge of your health journey with confidence, resilience, and unwavering determination.

Empowering Your Culinary Legacy

As you embark on this transformative culinary voyage towards optimal diverticulitis management, remember that you are crafting more than just delectable meals – you are weaving a legacy of health, vitality, and resilience for yourself and future generations. Each recipe you prepare, each meal you savor, becomes a testament to your commitment to nurturing your well-being and embracing a balanced, enjoyable diet that supports your health goals. By empowering yourself through the culinary mastery you cultivate, you leave behind a legacy of culinary wisdom and well-being that resonates far beyond the confines of your kitchen, inspiring others to embark on their own journey towards digestive wellness and culinary fulfillment.

Through the artful integration of knowledge, creativity, and culinary mastery, you can pave a path towards optimal diverticulitis management that is as enriching as it is empowering. As you embrace the transformative potential of diverticulitis-conscious cooking, remember that each meal you prepare is a testament to your commitment to health, well-being, and self-care. By nurturing your body with nourishing, flavorful dishes that cater to your specific dietary needs, you reclaim control over your health journey, reducing anxiety, empowering your culinary creativity, and savoring each meal as a celebration of vitality and resilience. Embrace the culinary adventure that lies ahead with confidence and enthusiasm, knowing that each dish you craft is a step towards a balanced, enjoyable diet that supports your health goals and enhances your overall well-being. In the tapestry of diverticulitis management, your culinary journey is a testament to your dedication to health, vitality, and culinary creativity, inspiring you to savor each meal as a masterpiece of well-being and empowerment.

Made in United States
Orlando, FL
02 December 2024

54868862R00059